Gourmet Keto Diet Cookbook

For Women After 50

150+ Tasty Low-Carb Recipes to Reverse Aging, Burn Fat and Boost Your Metabolism. Forget Digestive Problems, Acid Reflux and Be Super-Energetic

By

Serena Green

Table of Contents

Introduction

If you're just a woman over 50 years of age, you may be much more involved in weight loss than you would have been at 30. Most women face a slower metabolism at this age at a rate of around 50 calories a day. A slower metabolism will make it incredibly difficult to control weight gain, along with reduced exercise, muscle degradation, and the propensity for increased hunger pangs. There are several diet options available to help lose weight, but the keto diet is amongst the most famous lately. The keto diet (or ketogenic diet, for short) is indeed a low-carb, high-fat diet that promises numerous health benefits. We have obtained several questions about keto's feasibility and how to adapt the diet in such a healthier way. More than 20 studies have shown that sort of diet can lead to weight loss and health enhancement. Diabetes, cancer, epilepsy, and Alzheimer's can still benefit from ketogenic diets. To make the body burn its very own fat stores more effectively, Keto is a diet that involves reducing carbohydrates and growing fats. Analysis has also shown that a keto diet is suitable for general health and weight reduction. In particular, ketogenic diets have enabled certain individuals to lose excess body fat without the extreme hunger pangs characteristic of most diets. Any patients with type 2 diabetes have also been shown to be able to use keto to manage their signs. At the core of a ketogenic diet are ketones. As an alternative energy source, the body creates ketones, a fuel molecule, while getting short on blood sugar. When you decrease carb consumption and eat only the proper levels of nutrients, ketone production happens. Your liver will convert body ketones when you consume keto-friendly foods, which are then used by your body as an energy supply. You are in ketosis as the body uses fat for energy supply. This causes the body, in some situations, to dramatically increase its fat burning, which helps to minimize pockets of excess fat. This fat-burning approach not only lets you lose some weight, but it could also fend off cravings during the day and eliminate sugar crashes. While it's straightforward to assume that the keto diet is high in fat and low in carbohydrates, while you're in the supermarket aisle, it still feels a little more complicated. If Keto is right for you or not depends on several variables. A ketogenic diet can have many advantages, especially for weight loss, providing you don't suffer from health problems. Eating a perfect mix of greens, lean beef, and unrefined carbohydrates are the most significant thing to note. It is possible that keeping the whole foods is the most successful way to eat healthily, mainly because it is a sustainable strategy. It is important to remember that a lot of literature suggests that it is impossible to continue with ketogenic diets. For this cause, discovering a safe eating plan that appeals to you is the right advice. It's cool to try good experiences, but don't leap headfirst. If you are a female over 50 and want to change your lifestyle, this book will teach you what you need to learn about the keto diet. Breakfast, lunch, dinner recipes, and some tasty keto snacks and smoothie recipes are tasty, convenient, and straightforward to make for you. To sustain a balanced lifestyle after 50, let's just begin reading.

Chapter 1: The Keto Diet: A Better Way Towards Improved Health for Women Over 50

1.1. Keto diet in a nutshell

The keto diet is a high-fat, low-carbohydrate diet similar to Atkins & low-carb diets. It involves substantially reducing the consumption of carbohydrates and replacing them with fat. "Ketogenic" is a low-carb food idea (like the Atkins diet). The idea is to get more calories from proteins, fats, and less from carbohydrates. One has to remove carbohydrates such as starch, soda, pastry, and white bread, which are simple to digest. This reduction in calories takes the body to a regular cycle of the body, which is called ketosis. When this happens, the liver is extremely energy efficient when processing fat. It also transforms fat into ketones in the liver that can supply energy to the brain. Ketogenic diets can contribute to substantial decreases in blood sugar and insulin levels. This, combined with the increased ketones, has a range of health effects. If you eat less than 50 grams of carbohydrate a day, your body will eventually run out of fuel (sugar in your blood) and eat it easily. It normally takes about 3 and 4 days. Then you start to break down protein and energy fat that can help you drop weight. It's referred to as ketosis. It is necessary to note that the ketogenic diet is not about dietary benefits, but rather about a short-term diet that focuses on weight loss. People use ketogenic diets to lose weight most frequently, although they may also help to address certain medical problems, including epilepsy. People with heart disease, brain diseases, and even acne can benefit, but more research in these fields is required. First, talk to your doctor about whether a ketogenic diet is healthy, particularly if you have type 1 diabetes.

1.2. Yes, keto is fine for women over 50

There are certain common dangers and issues that relate to anyone who consumes keto, such as the need to add electrolytes to prevent cramps. It's crucial for anyone to grasp the diet and do it appropriately. Especially for women above 50, it could mean paying particular attention to calcium or making sure they have enough food to remain well-nourished. There are still individuals — both men and women — who simply don't work on low-carb diets for a particular reason, and that's all right.

Some several unique concerns and subjects relate mainly or exclusively to women. Yet overall, there is very little proof that healthy women who are just not pregnant may be more worried about keto than some other diet. There is no proof that people necessarily cannot or cannot consume keto – in fact, there are many women who do keto and enjoy keto! And there is also some proof that keto diets can be beneficial to some female-specific problems, such as PCOS.'

1.3. Key takeaways for women above 50 on keto Diet

o   Get the correct protein quantity

o   Don't eat far too much fat.

o   fast intermittently

o   Look out for the creeping carb

o   Cut the alcohol out

o   Evite the sweeteners

o   Do a weightlifting workout

o   Get ample sleep right now

o   Reducing tension

o   Be rational about this

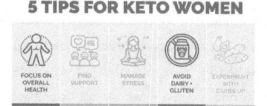

1.4. Problems to be aware of regarding keto diet in over 50 women

One issue that women can face with keto diets about the under-eating to the extent of a physically unsafe energy deficiency or a lack of body fat underneath a safe amount. It's quite likely to consume less on keto, deliberately or accidentally. Many people who pursue keto seem to be healthy-conscious individuals who want to exercise out a lot, which only increases the issue when they consume less, then drives themselves into intense exercises that need more protein and calories to recover.

This is much more harmful to women than for men since the female body is vulnerable to malnutrition. The reduction of bone mass, a higher likelihood of bone stress fractures, a higher risk of anemia, stomach issues, and psychiatric symptoms.

Dieting to the extent of missing your time can even happen without some workout at all, and it's almost as risky that way! Nutrition Disease

None of this is special to keto. It's all like the calorie deficit. But the appetizing benefits of keto diet increase the risks that women attempting to lose weight will not know how severe they are, mainly because they'll actually receive nothing but compliments about how "safe" they're eating and how "sweet" they're consuming absolutely nothing.

Although, of course, the repression of hunger often renders the diet appealing to women living with eating disorders. It's not exactly a "keto danger;" it's a danger of violating keto, but it does occur. It's outside the meaning of a single post to really consider coping with it, so it sounds like someone you meet, reach out to — you could be saving a life.

Chapter 2: Keto Breakfast recipes for women over 50

Let's be realistic; one of life's biggest pleasures is a carbohydrate-rich breakfast. There are plenty of safe and tasty keto-friendly breakfast meals. And there is a lot you're probably going to save them from trying someday.

1. Keto Hot chocolate shake

Servings: 1 cup | Total time: 10 min

Calories: 193 | Proteins: 2g | Carbohydrates: 4 g | Fat: 18g

Ingredients

○ Two tablespoons unsweetened cocoa powder
○ Two and a half teaspoon sugar
○ One-fourth cup of water
○ One-fourth cup heavy cream
○ One-fourth teaspoon pure vanilla extract
○ Some whipped cream, for the purpose of serving

Steps of preparation

○ In a medium bowl on medium-low heat, mix together chocolate, swerve, and around two tablespoons of water until everything is smooth and absorbed. Increase down to a simmer, introduce remaining water & cream, and periodically whisk until heated.
○ Stir in the vanilla, and dump in the cup. Start serving with whipped cream or chocolate powder.

2. Keto delicious Cereal

Servings: 3 cups | Total time: 35 min

Calories: 188 | Proteins: 4g | Carbohydrates: 7 g | Fat: 17g

Ingredients

○ Cooking spray
○ One cup almond, chopped walnuts
○ One fourth cup sesame seeds
○ Coconut flakes
○ Two tablespoon flax seeds
○ Two tablespoon chia seeds
○ Half teaspoon ground clove
○ One and a half teaspoon ground cinnamon
○ One teaspoon pure vanilla extract
○ Half teaspoon kosher salt
○ One large egg white
○ One-fourth cup melted coconut oil

Steps of preparation

○ Preheat the oven to 350 ° C then oil the baking tray with a cooking spray. In a wide cup, add coconut flakes, almonds, sesame seeds, walnuts, and chia seeds and linseeds Stir with garlic, vanilla, salt, and cinnamon,

o   Now Beat the egg white into foamy and mix in the granola. Apply the coconut oil and mix until all is well covered. Pour over the baking tray and scatter over a consistent layer. Bake for 20 mins just until it gets crispy, stirring gently halfway through. Let it just to cool completely.

3. Keto Sausage Sandwich

Servings: 3 | Total time: 15 min

Calories: 411 | Proteins: 38g | Carbohydrates: 7.3 g | Fat: 27g

Ingredients

o   Six large eggs
o   Two tablespoons heavy cream
o   Pinch of red pepper flakes
o   Pinch of Kosher salt
o   Three slices cheddar
o   Six frozen sausage patties
o   Freshly ground black pepper
o   One teaspoon butter
o   Avocado in sliced pieces

Steps of preparation

o   Beat the eggs, red pepper flakes, and heavy cream in a shallow cup. Season to taste with salt carefully. Melt the butter in

a non - stick pan over medium heat. In the bowl, pour approximately 1/3 of the whites. Place the cheese mostly in center and then let it rest for around 1 minute. Place the corners of the egg in the center, shielding the cheese. Remove from heat and perform the same on remaining eggs.

o   Serve the eggs in two avocado sausage patties.

4. Ketogenic Cabbage Hash Browns

Servings: 2 | Total time: 10 min

Calories: 230 | Proteins: 8g | Carbohydrates: 6 g | Fat: 19g

Ingredients

o   Two large eggs
o   Half teaspoon garlic powder
o   Half teaspoon kosher salt
o   Grounded black pepper
o   Two cups shredded cabbage
o   One fourth small yellow onion
o   One tablespoon vegetable oil

Steps of preparation

o   In a big cup, mix together eggs, salt and garlic. Season with salt and pepper. Apply the cabbage and the onion to the beaten egg and mix to blend.

o   Heat the oil skillet over medium-high flame. Roughly divide the prepared mixture into four patties in the skillet and pressure the spatula to compress. Cook until yellow golden and juicy.

5. Ketogenic Pancakes for breakfast

Servings: 6 | Total time: 15 min

Calories: 268 | Proteins: 9g | Carbohydrates: 6 g | Fat: 23g

Ingredients

o Half cup almond flour
o Four oz. cream cheese
o Four large eggs
o One teaspoon lemon zest
o Butter

Steps of preparation

o In a medium cup, blend together the rice, the eggs, the cream cheese, and the lemon zest until soft and smooth.
o Melt 1 tablespoon of butter on medium heat in a frying pan. Pour in approximately 3 teaspoons of the batter and simmer for 2 minutes until golden. Flip and cook for 2 more minutes. Move to the plate and continue for the remainder of the batter.
o Serve with some sugar and butter.

6. Keto breakfast quick Smoothie

Servings: 6 | Total time: 5 min

Calories: 152 | Proteins: 1g | Carbohydrates: 5 g | Fat: 13g

Ingredients

o One and a half cup frozen strawberries
o One and a half cup frozen raspberries, plus more for garnish (optional)
o One cup frozen blackberry
o Two cup coconut milk
o One cup baby spinach
o Shaved coconut for garnishing purposes

Steps of preparation

o Combine all the ingredients (except coconut) in a mixer. Mix so that it gets creamy.
o Divide, if used, into cups and top with raspberries and coconut.

7. Keto Breakfast Cups

Servings: 12 cups | Total time: 40 min

Calories: 82 kcal | Proteins: 6g | Carbohydrates: 1 g | Fat: 2g

Ingredients

o Two pounds ground pork
o Two tablespoon freshly chopped thyme
o Two cloves of minced garlic
o Half teaspoon paprika
o Half teaspoon. ground cumin
o One teaspoon kosher salt
o Half cup ground black pepper.
o One cup chopped fresh spinach
o White cheddar shredded

- o Twelve eggs
- o One tablespoon freshly chopped chive

Steps of preparation

- o Start by preheating the oven to 400 ° F. Mix the ground pork, garlic, paprika, thyme, salt and the cumin in a large dish. Now season with a salt and the pepper.
- o Add just that small handful of pork per muffin container, and then push the sides to create a cup. Start dividing spinach and cheese similarly in cups. Crack the egg at the top of every cup and add salt and pepper for seasoning.

8. Keto Breakfast Blueberry Muffins

Servings: 12 muffins | Total time: 40 min

Calories: 181 kcal | Proteins: 4.5g | Carbohydrates: 25 g | Fat: 5.6g

Ingredients

- o Two and a half cup almond flour
- o One third cup keto friendly sugar
- o One and a half teaspoon baking powder
- o Half teaspoon baking soda
- o Half teaspoon kosher salt
- o One-third cup melted butter
- o One-third cup unsweetened almond milk
- o Three large eggs
- o One teaspoon pure vanilla extract
- o Two-third cup blueberries
- o Half lemon zests

Steps of preparation

- o Start by preheating the oven to a temperature of 350 ° and put in a muffin tray with cupcake liners.
- o In a big container, stir together almond flour, Swerve, baking soda, baking powder, and salt. Gently stir in melted butter, eggs, and vanilla once mixed.
- o Gently fold the blueberries and the lemon zest until uniformly spread. Scoop equivalent quantities of the mixture into each liner of cupcakes and bake until softly golden and a toothpick inserted into the middle of the muffin comes out clean, this will happen within 23 minutes. Let it cool slightly before serving.

9. Keto Thai Beef Lettuce Wraps

Serving: 4| Total Time: 30 min|

Calories: 368 Kcal, Fat: 14.5g, Net Carbs: 3.1g, Protein: 53.8g

Ingredients

- o Olive oil 1 tablespoon
- o Ground beef 1.5lb.
- o Beef stock 1 ½ cups
- o Garlic 2 cloves, minced
- o lime juice fresh ¼ cup
- o Fish sauce 2 tablespoons
- o Chopped parsley ½ cup
- o Mint chopped ½ cup

o To taste salt & pepper

Steps of Preparation

o Heat the olive oil over medium to high heat in a skillet.

o In a skillet, brown the beef for eight to ten mins.

o Add beef to skillet.

o Cook till the stock has fully boiled off.

o Meanwhile, mix the garlic, fish sauce, and lime juice.

o Add beef to the lime mixture.

o Cook 2 to 3 mins.

o Garnish with chopped herbs.

o Assemble, the beef is scooped over the leaves of the cabbage or the lettuce.

o Serve.

10. Breakfast Skillet Cilantro-Lime Chicken

Serving 4 | Total Time: 30 min

Calories: Kcal 426, Fat: 16.4g, Net Carbs: 6g, Protein: 61.8g

Ingredients

o Olive oil 1 tbsp

o Chicken breasts 4 boneless skinless

o Kosher salt

o Ground freshly black pepper

o Unsalted butter 2 tbsp

o Garlic minced 2 cloves

o Medium limes 2 finely grated zest

o Lime juice freshly squeezed 1/4 cup

o Freshly chopped cilantro leaves & tender stems 1/3 cup

o (Optional) for serving cooked rice

Steps of Preparation

o Pat the chicken, thoroughly dry using paper towels. Season properly with pepper and salt. Steam 1 tbsp of the oil over medium to high shimmering steam in a ten-inch or bigger skillet. If possible, working in batches, add the chicken and sear to the bottom for 5 to 7 minutes, until deeply browned. Flip the meat, then sear for 5 to 7 mins before the other side is browned. Place the chicken into a plate; put aside.

o Reduce to medium heat. Attach the garlic, butter, and lime zest then cook for 1 minute, stirring frequently. Stir in the juice of the lime. Send the chicken back to the skillet and any leftover juices. Cover, heat is reduced as required to maintain a moderate simmer and cook till the meat is cooked through and record 165°F on thermometer instant-read, 2 to 3 min.

o Stir some of the sauce and the cilantro and pour over the chicken. When desired, eat with rice.

11. Breakfast keto Buffalo Chicken

Serving 4-6 | Total Time: 29 min

Calories: 295 Kcal, Fat: 12.6g, Net Carbs: 0g, Protein: 42.6g

Ingredients

- Boneless chicken breasts 2 1/2 pounds skinless
- Bottle hot sauce 1 (12-ounce)
- Ghee or unsalted butter 4 tbsp

Steps of Preparation

- In a 6-quarter or Electric Pressure Cooker, bigger Instant Pot put 2 1/2 pounds of chicken breasts boneless, skinless into one layer. Pour 1 (12-ounce) spicy chicken sauce bottle over it. Cube 4 tbsp of ghee or unsalted butter, then put the chicken on top.
- Lock the cover in place and ensure that the valve is shut. High pressure cooking to cook about 15 minutes. It's going to take 10 - 12 minutes to work up under pressure. Once the time for cooking is finished, let the pressure drop for 5 min naturally. Release the remaining pressure
- Move the chicken right away to a clean cutting plate. For slice the meat, using two forks, then move to a dish. Whisk the sauce once mixed and emulsified in a pressure cooker. Apply to chicken 1 cup sauce and flip to coat. Apply more sauce if appropriate and set aside any leftover sauce to consume or store.

12. Chocolate Breakfast Keto Protein Shake

Servings: 1 | Total time: 40 min

Calories: 445 kcal | Proteins: 31g | Carbohydrates: 7 g | Fat: 12g

Ingredients

- Three fourth cup almond milk
- Half cup ices
- Two tablespoon almond butter
- Two tablespoons unsweetened cocoa powder
- Two tablespoons keto-friendly sugar
- One tablespoon chia seed
- Two tablespoon hemp seeds
- Half table pure vanilla extract
- A Pinch of kosher salt

Steps of preparation

- Mix all ingredients together in a blender and process until smooth. Pour in a bowl and compote with a little more chia & hemp seeds.

13. Breakfast Bell Pepper Eggs

Servings: 3 yields | Total time: 20 min

Calories: 121 kcal | Proteins: 8.6g | Carbohydrates: 4 g | Fat: 7.9g

Ingredients

- One bell pepper

- Six eggs
- Pinch kosher salt
- Pinch of freshly ground black peppers
- Two tablespoon chopped chives
- Two tablespoon chopped parsley

Steps of preparation

- Warm a nonstick saucepan over medium heat then gently oil with a cooking mist.
- Place the bell pepper ring in the pan and simmer for 2 minutes. Swap the ring, then break the egg there in the middle of it. Add salt and pepper, then simmer until the egg is prepared to your preference for two to four minutes.
- Repeat the same procedure with other eggs and serve with the chives and the parsley.

14. Omelet-Stuffed Peppers

Servings: 4 | Total time: 1 hour

Calories: 380 kcal | Proteins: 26g | Carbohydrates: 4.5 g | Fat: 28g

Ingredients

- Two bell peppers
- Eight eggs
- One fourth cup milk
- Four slices of bacon cooked
- One cup shredded cheddar
- Two tablespoon finely chopped chives
- A pinch of Kosher salt

- Black pepper crushed

Steps of preparation

- Preheat the oven to 400 ° C. Now place the peppers sliced horizontally in a big baking sheet. Apply a very little water to the sheet and bake the pepper for five minutes.
- In the meanwhile, beat the eggs and milk together. Stir in sausage, cheese, and chips and add salt and pepper as required.
- When the peppers are baked, apply the egg mixture to the peppers. Place in the oven and cook for 35 to 40 minutes until the eggs have been set. Garnish with a little more chives and eat.

15. Keto breakfast Clouded Bread

Servings: 6 rolls | Total time: 35 min

Calories: 98 kcal | Proteins: 4g | Carbohydrates: 0.2 g | Fat: 9g

Ingredients

- Three large eggs
- One fourth teaspoon cream of tartar
- A Pinch of kosher salt
- Two oz. cream cheese
- One tablespoon Italian seasoning
- One tablespoon shredded mozzarella
- Two teaspoon tomato paste
- Pinch of kosher salt

- One teaspoon poppy seed
- One teaspoon sesame seed
- One teaspoon minced dried garlic
- One teaspoon minced dried onion

Steps of preparation

- Start by preheating the oven to 300 ° C and cover a wide pan with parchment paper.

- Separate the egg whites from its yolks in 2 small glass containers. Apply the cream of the tartar and the salt to the egg whites, then with a hand blender, beat until solid. It will happen within 2 to 3 minutes. Transfer the cream cheese to the egg yolks and now, using a hand blender, combine the yolks and the cream cheese until blended. Gently incorporate the egg yolk mixture in the egg whites.

- Divide the dough into portions of 8 mounds on a lined baking sheet, 4 "off from each other—Bake until it becomes golden, which will happen within twenty-five to thirty minutes.

- Instantly sprinkle each slice of bread with cheese and oven for two or three minutes. Let it cool a bit. Easy plain cloud bread is ready for you.

- Add 1 tablespoon of Italian seasoning, two tablespoons of shredded mozzarella or parmesan cheese, and two tablespoons

of tomato paste to the egg yolk mixture. Add 1 tablespoon of Italian seasoning, two tablespoons of shredded mozzarella or parmesan cheese, and two tablespoons of tomato paste to the egg yolk mixture. Bake until it becomes golden, which will happen within twenty-five to thirty minutes.

- Add 1/8 teaspoon of kosher salt, 1 teaspoon of poppy seeds, 1 teaspoon of sesame seeds, 1 teaspoon of mashed dried garlic, then 1 teaspoon of chopped dried onion to the egg yolk mixture. (Or use 1 tablespoon with all bagel seasoning.) All bagel cloud bread is set.

- Add 1 1/2 teaspoons of ranch seasoning powder to the egg mixture. Bake until it becomes golden, which will happen within twenty-five to thirty minutes. Ranch cloud bread is ready to go.

16. Breakfast Jalapeño Popper Egg Cups

Servings: 12 cups | Total time: 1 hour

Calories: 157.2kcal | Proteins: 9.5 g | Carbohydrates: 1.3 g | Fat: 12.2 g

Ingredients

- Twelve slices bacon
- Ten large eggs
- One fourth cup sour cream

- Half cup shredded Cheddar
- Half cup shredded mozzarella
- Two jalapeños, one minced and one thinly sliced
- One teaspoon garlic powder
- A pinch of kosher salt
- Cooking spray
- Ground black pepper

Steps of preparation

- Preheat the oven to 375 ° C. Cook the bacon in a wide medium saucepan until it is well golden brown and still stackable. To drain, put aside on a paper towel-lined dish to drain.
- In a large plastic container, stir together eggs, cheese, sour cream, jalapeno minced, and garlic powder. Season to taste with salt & pepper.
- Use a nonstick cooking spray to oil the muffin tin. Fill each well along with one slice of bacon, then add the egg mixture into each muffin tin until around two-thirds of the way to the tin's top   Cover each muffin with a slice of jalapeno.
- Bake for a period of 20 minutes just until the eggs are no longer sticky. Cool briefly before withdrawing the muffin tin.

17. Keto Zucchini Breakfast Egg Cups

Servings: 18 cups | Total time: 35 min

Calories: 17   kcal | Proteins: 1   g | Carbohydrates: 1.3 g | Fat: 1 g

Ingredients

- Cooking spray
- Two zucchinis peeled
- One fourth lb. ham
- Half cup cherry tomatoes
- Eight eggs
- Half cup heavy cream
- A pinch of Kosher salt
- A grounded black pepper
- Half teaspoon dried oregano
- One Pinch red pepper flakes
- One cup shredded cheddar

Steps of preparation

- Start by preheating the oven to 400 ° F and oil the muffin tray with a cooking mist. To form a crust, line inside and underside of muffin tin with both the zucchini strips. Sprinkle with the cherry tomatoes and the ham each crust.
- In a medium container, stir together eggs, whipping cream, oregano & red pepper flakes and add salt and pepper. Pour the egg mixture over the ham and tomatoes and cover with the cheese.
- Bake for 30 minutes until eggs are ready.

18. Breakfast Brussels Sprouts Hash

Servings: 4 cups | Total time: 40 min

Calories: 181 kcal | Proteins: 3 g | Carbohydrates: 13 g | Fat: 14 g

Ingredients

o Six slices bacon
o Half chopped onion
o One lb. Brussels
o An inch of Kosher salt
o Black pepper grounded
o One fourth teaspoon crushed red pepper flakes
o Two minced cloves garlic
o Four large eggs

Steps of preparation

o Cook bacon until crispy in a large frying pan. Switch off the heat and move the bacon to a paper towel tray. Hold much of the bacon fat in the pan, cut some black specks from the pan.

o Turn the heat down to low and transfer the onion and Brussels to the pan. Cook, stirring regularly before vegetables start to turn soft and turn golden. Season to taste with salt, pepper & red pepper flakes.

o Transfer 2 tablespoons of water in the mixture and cover the pan. Cook till the Brussels are soft, and the water gets evaporated for about five minutes. (If all the water is gone until the sprouts are soft, add a little more water to the pan and cover for a few more minutes.) Put the garlic to the pan. Cook until fragrant for almost 1 minute.

o Cut four holes in the hash using a wooden spoon, to expose the base of the pan. Break an egg into each gap and add salt and pepper for each egg. Replace the lid and cook it until eggs are ready to your taste, which is around 5 minutes for the egg that is runny

o Sprinkle the cooked bacon bites over the whole pan and serve hot.

19. Best Breakfast Keto Bread

Servings: 1 bread | Total time: 40 min

Calories: 165 kcal | Proteins: 6 g | Carbohydrates: 3 g | Fat: 15 g

Ingredients

o One fourth cup butter, melted and cooled
o One and a half cup ground almond
o Six large eggs
o Half teaspoon cream of tartar
o One tablespoon baking powder
o Half teaspoon kosher salt

Steps of preparation

o Start by preheating the oven to 375 ° F and then line the 8"-x-4 "loaf on a baking sheet. Completely separate egg whites from egg yolk.

- In a wide container, mix egg whites with tarter cream. Using a hand blender, keep whipping until strong peaks are created.

- Shake the yolks with melted butter, baking powder, almond flour, and salt in a separate big bowl using a hand blender. Fold in 1/3 of egg whites when completely blended, then fold in the remainder.

- Load the batter into the loaf pan and make flat layer. Then Bake for 30 minutes or until the surface is softly golden, and the toothpick comes out clean. Enable to cool for 30 minutes before cutting.

20. Bacon Breakfast Avocado Bombs

Servings: 4 bombs | Total time: 25 min

Calories: 251 kcal | Proteins: 6 g | Carbohydrates: 13 g | Fat: 18 g

Ingredients

- Two avocados
- One-third shredded Cheddar
- Eight slices bacon

Steps of preparation

- Steam the broiler and line up a narrow baking sheet with foil.

- Cut each avocado into half and scrape the pits. Take the skin off from each of the avocados.

- Cover two-thirds of the cheese, and substitute with the other thirds of the avocado. Cover 4 pieces of bacon in each avocado.

- Put the bacon-wrapped avocados upon this lined baking sheet and broil till the bacon is crisp, approximately 5 minutes. Turn the avocado really carefully and proceed to cook till crispy all around, approximately five minutes per side.

- Break half lengthwise and serve instantly.

21. Breakfast Ham & Cheese keto Egg Cups

Servings: 12 cups | Total time: 35 min

Calories: 108 kcal | Proteins: 10.4 g | Carbohydrates: 1.2 g | Fat: 5.9 g

Ingredients

- Cooking spray
- Twelve slices of ham
- One cup shredded cheddar
- Twelve large eggs
- A pinch of Kosher salt
- Ground black pepper
- Parsley, for garnish

Steps of preparation

- Preheat the oven to 400o and oil the 12-cup muffin tray with a cooking mist. Top each cup with just a piece of ham and top with cheddar. Break an egg inside each ham cup and add salt and pepper.

o Bake until the eggs are roasted thru, 12 to 15 minutes.

o Garnish with parsley, serve.

22. Keto Breakfast Peanut Fat Bombs

Servings: 12 bombs | Total time: 1 hour 40 min

Calories: 247 kcal | Proteins: 3.6 g | Carbohydrates: 3.3 g | Fat: 24.4 g

Ingredients

o Eight oz. cream cheese
o A pinch of kosher salt
o Half cup dark chocolate chips
o Half cup peanut butter
o One fourth cup coconut oil

Steps of preparation

o Line a narrow baking sheet with a sheet of parchment paper. In a medium container, mix cream cheese with peanut butter, 1/4 cup of coconut oil, and some salt. Using a hand blender, beat the mixture until it becomes thoroughly mixed, approximately for 2 minutes. Put the bowl in the freezer until it is lightly firmed, for 10 to 15 minutes.

o When a peanut butter mixture is formed, use a tiny cookie scoop to produce spoonful-sized balls. Put in the refrigerator for 5 minutes to harden.

o In the meantime, produce a chocolate drizzle by mixing chocolate chips and the leftover coconut oil in a large mixing bowl and microwave it for 30 seconds until completely melted. Drizzle over the balls of peanut butter and then put in the refrigerator for 5 minutes.

o Keep wrapped in the refrigerator to stock.

23. Breakfast keto Paleo Stacks

Servings: 3 | Total time: 30 min

Calories: 229 kcal | Proteins: 3 g | Carbohydrates: 11 g | Fat: 18 g

Ingredients

o Three sausage patties
o One mashed avocado
o A pinch of kosher salt
o Ground black pepper
o Three large eggs
o Hot sauce as required

Steps of preparation

o Heat the breakfast sausage.

o Mash the avocado onto the breakfast sausage and add salt and pepper.

o Spray a medium pan over medium heat with only a cooking spray and then spray the interior of the mason jar cap. Place the mason jar lid within middle of the pan and break the egg inside. Add salt and pepper and cook for 3 minutes until hot, then remove the cover and continue to cook.

o Place the egg on top of the mashed avocado. Season with chives and sleet with the hot sauce you want.

24. Breakfast keto quick chaffles

Servings: 2 yields | Total time: 25 min

Calories: 115 kcal | Proteins: 9 g | Carbohydrates: 1 g | Fat: 8 g

Ingredients

o Four eggs
o 8 oz. shredded cheddar cheese
o Two tablespoon chives
o A pinch of salt and pepper
o 4 eggs for toppings
o Eight bacons
o Eight cherry tomatoes diced
o Two oz. baby spinach

Steps of preparation

o Organize the bacon slices in a big, unheated pan and set the temperature to moderate flame. Golden brown the bacon for 8-12 mins, turning often, until crispy to bite.

o Put aside on a paper towel to drain when you're cooking.
o Put all of the waffle ingredients in a mixing container and blend well.
o Lightly oil the waffle iron and afterward uniformly spoon the mixture over the bottom of the tray, spreading it out gently to achieve even outcomes.
o Shut the waffle iron and cook for roughly. 6 minutes, depending on capacity of the waffle maker.
o Crack an egg in the bacon fat in the cooking pan and cook slowly until finished.
o Serve each tablespoon of scrambled egg and bacon pieces along with some baby spinach and some sliced cherry tomatoes.

25. Keto breakfast with fried eggs, tomato, and cheese

Total Time: 15 mins |Serving 1

Calories: Kcal 417, Fat:33g, Net Carbs:4g Protein:25g

Ingredients

o Eggs 2
o Butter ½ tbsp
o Cubed cheddar cheese 2 oz
o Tomato ½
o Ground black pepper & salt

Steps of Preparation

- Heat butter over medium heat in a frying pan.
- Season the diced side of the tomato with salt & pepper. Put the tomato in a frying pan.
- Break the eggs in the same pan. Leaving the eggs to scramble on one side for eggs sunny side up. Rotate the eggs for a couple of mins and cook for one more minute for eggs fried over quickly. Cook for a few more minutes for tougher yolks. Season with salt & pepper.
- On a plate, Put the eggs, tomatoes, and cheese to eat. Scatter with dried oregano eggs and tomatoes for some additional flavor and taste.

26. Keto eggs Benedict on avocado

Total Time: 15 mins | Serving 4

Calories: Kcal 522, Fat:48g, Net Carbs:3g Protein:16g

Ingredients

Hollandaise

- Egg yolks 3
- Lemon juice 1 tbsp
- Salt & pepper
- Unsalted butter 8½ tbsp

Eggs benedict

- Pitted & skinned avocados 2
- Eggs 4
- Smoked salmon 5 oz

Steps of Preparation

- Take a mason jar or other microwave-safe containers that will fit easily inside the immersion blender. Put the butter and then melt for around 20 seconds in the microwave.
- In butter, incorporate the yolks of egg and lemon juice. The hand blender is Placed at the container bottom and combine until a creamy white coating is created. Raise the blender and lower it slowly to create a creamy sauce.
- Place a saucepan over the stove with water and boil. Decrease the heat to low.
- Crack the eggs, one at a time, in a cup, and then carefully slip each into the bowl. Stirring the water in a circle can keep the egg white from displacing too much from the yolk. Cook 3-4 mins, depending on the yolk quality you like. To retain excess water, remove the eggs with a spoon.
- Break the avocados in two and remove the skin and stones. Create a slice of each half around the base, so it rests equally on the dish. Cover with one egg every half, then finish with a hollandaise sauce

generous dollop. Load some smoked salmon.

o This dish must be consumed promptly and should not preserve or reheat. Hollandaise sauce Leftover can be preserved for up to 4 days in a fridge.

27. Keto quick low carb mozzarella chaffles

Total Time: 8 mins | Serving 4

Calories: Kcal 330, Fat:27g, Net Carbs:2g Protein:20g

Ingredients

o Melted butter 1 oz.
o Eggs 4
o Shredded mozzarella cheese 8 oz
o Almond flour 4 tbsp

Steps of Preparation

o Heat the waffle maker.
o Put all of the ingredients in a mixing bowl and beat to blend.
o Lightly oil the waffle iron with the butter, then spoon the mixture uniformly over the bottom, spreading it out to achieve an even outcome. Cover the waffle iron, then cook depending on the waffle maker, for approx. 6 mins.
o Release the cap softly when you feel it's done.
o Serve with favorite toppings.

28. Nut-free keto bread

Total Time: 50 mins | Serving 20

Calories: Kcal 105, Fat:8g, Net Carbs:1g Protein:6g

Ingredients

o Eggs 6
o Shredded cheese 12 oz
o Cream cheese 1 oz
o Husk powder ground psyllium 2 tbsp
o Baking powder 3 tsp
o Oat fiber ½ cup
o Salt ½ tsp
o Melted butter 1 tbsp

Topping

o Sesame seeds 3 tbsp
o Poppy seeds 2 tbsp

Steps of Preparation

o To 180 ° C (360 ° F), preheat the oven.
o Whisk eggs. Attach the cheese and the other ingredients, except the butter, and stir properly.
o Grease a buttered bread pan (8.5 " x 4.5 "x 2.75," non-stick or parchment-papered). Spread the dough with a spatula in the bread-pan.
o Sprinkle with poppy and sesame seeds over the rice. 35 Mins to bake the loaf.
o Let cool down the bread.

29. Simple keto breakfast with fried eggs

Total Time: 10 mins | Serving 1

Calories: Kcal 425, Fat:41g, Net Carbs:1g Protein:13g

Ingredients

o Eggs 2

o Butter 1 tbsp

o Mayonnaise 2 tbsp

o Baby spinach 1 oz

o Ground black pepper & salt

o Coffee or tea 1 cup

Steps of Preparation

o Heat butter over med heat in a frying pan.

o Crack the eggs into the pan right away. For sunny side up eggs, -leaving one side of the eggs to fry. Cooked over quick for eggs-flip over the eggs after a couple of mins and cook for 1 more minute. Only stop the cooking for a few more mins for stronger yolks. Season with pepper and salt

o Serve a dollop of mayonnaise with baby spinach.

2.30. Keto taco omelet

Total Time: 20 mins | Serving 2

Calories: Kcal 797, Fat:63g, Net Carbs:8g Protein:44g

Ingredients

Taco seasoning

o Onion powder ¼ tsp

o Ground cumin ½ tsp

o Paprika powder ½ tsp

o Garlic powder ½ tsp

o Chili flakes ¼ tsp

o Salt ½ tsp

o Ground black pepper ¼ tsp

o Fresh oregano ½ tsp

Omelet

o Ground beef 5 oz

o Large eggs 4

o Olive oil 1 tbsp

o Avocado 1

o Shredded cheddar cheese 5 oz

o Diced tomato 1

o Fresh cilantro 1 tsp

o Sea salt ½ tsp

o Ground black pepper ¼ tsp

Steps of Preparation

o Combine all Taco Seasoning products.

o In a large non-stick pan, add the ground beef. Apply the seasoning mixture(taco), blend well, and fry till completely cooked. Set aside in the bowl and remove it from heat.

- Beat the eggs in a mixing bowl and brush until they are soft.
- Reduce heat and add the olive oil in the saucepan. And add the eggs. Push the edges into the center, enabling the uncooked pieces to spill to the side, while the edges become solid. Cook a couple of mins, keep the inside a little runny.
- At ground beef, pinch lime.
- Break avocado half. The pit is Removed and suck the flesh out. Split into fragments.
- Spread ground beef over the omelet. Apply 2/3 of the grilled diced cheese and tomatoes.
- Remove the omelet cautiously from the pan. Add more avocado, cheese, and cilantro. Season salt & pepper. Serve.

30. Keto dosa

Total Time: 25 mins | Serving 2

Calories: Kcal 356, Fat:33g, Net Carbs:4g Protein:12g

Ingredients

- Almond flour ½ cup
- Shredded mozzarella cheese 1½ oz
- Coconut milk ½ cup
- Ground cumin ½ tsp
- Ground coriander seed ½ tsp
- Salt

Steps of Preparation

- Mix All ingredients in a bowl.
- Heat a non-stick skillet and oil lightly. The use of a non-stick skillet is very important to avoid the dosa from adhering to the pan.
- Pour in and spread the batter, by the pan moving.
- Cook on low heat the dosa. The cheese starts melting and crisping away.
- Once all the way through, it is cooked, and the dosa has turned golden brown on a side using the spatula fold it.
- Serve with chutney made from coconut.

For the Peanut Sauce:

- Peanut butter 1/2 cup
- Minced fresh ginger 1 tsp
- Minced fresh garlic 1 tsp
- Minced jalapeño pepper 1 Tbsp
- Sugar-free fish sauce 1 tbsp
- Sugar rice wine vinegar 2 tbsp
- Lime juice 1 tbsp
- Water 2 tbsp
- Erythritol granulated (sweetener) 2 tbsp

Steps of Preparation

For the Chicken:

- In a big bowl, Mix the fresh lemon juice, fish sauce, soy sauce, Rice vinegar,

28

avocado oil, cayenne pepper, ginger, garlic, ground coriander & sweetener, and whisk.

o Apply pieces of chicken and stir to thoroughly coat the chicken only with marinade.

o Cover & chill up to twenty-four hrs., or for at least 1 hr.

o Remove 1/2 hr. before cooking from the freezer & heat the grill.

o Grill the chicken on med heat for around 6 to 8 mins each side.

o Remove it from the grill, add peanut sauce & serve.

o Chopped up cabbage, diced peanuts, minced scallions & minced cilantro are optional garnishes.

For the Sauce with Peanut:

o Mix all the ingredients from the sauce in a mixer & mix till smooth.

o Before serving, taste and set sweetness& saltiness to your choice.

31. One-Skillet Chicken with Lemon Garlic Cream Sauce

Total Time: 30 mins |Serving 4|

Ingredients

o Skinless &boneless chicken thighs 4
o Salt & pepper
o Chicken broth 1 cup
o Lemon juice 2 tbsp
o Minced garlic 1 tbsp
o Red pepper flakes ½ tsp
o Olive oil 1 tbsp
o Finely diced shallots ⅓ cup
o Salted butter 2 tbsp
o Heavy cream ¼ cup
o Chopped parsley 2 tbsp

Steps of Preparation

o The thighs or chicken breasts are pounded into 1⁄2-inch thickness using a mallet. Sprinkle both sides of the chicken with a pinch of salt & pepper.

o Mix the chicken broth, juice of lemon, red pepper flakes, & garlic into a two-cup measuring cup.

o Place a rack in the bottom 3rd of your oven & preheat to 375of.

o Heat the olive oil on med-high heat in the big oven-safe pan. Apply the chicken & let it to brown for 2 to 3 mins each side. Unless the chicken isn't fully cooked, don't worry, finish it in your oven. Take the chicken off to a plate.

o Decrease the flame-med, apply the shallots & the chicken broth combination to the pan. Drag the bottom of the skillet with a whisk, so that all brown pieces are loosened. Kick up the heat back to med height and let the sauce come to low heat. Continue cooking the sauce for 10 to 15 mins, or till the sauce stays about 1/3 cup.

o Take from the flame whenever the sauce has thickened, then apply the butter & whisk till it fully melts. Apply the heavy whipping cream with the pan off flame, whisk in to mix. Place the pan on the flame for only thirty sec, Do NOT let the sauce boil. Take away from heat, apply the chicken back into the skillet & sprinkle the chicken over the sauce. Put the pan 5 to 8 mins in the oven, or till the chicken is fully cooked. Season with minced parsley or basil & serve hot with extra slices of lemon.

32. Low Carb Chicken Enchilada (Green) Cauliflower Casserole

Total Time: 45 mins | Serving 1

Calories: Cal 311, Fat:18g, Net Carbs:4g Protein:33g

Ingredients

o Frozen cauliflower florets 20 oz
o Softened cream cheese 4 oz
o Shredded cooked chicken 2 cups
o Salsa Verde ½ cups
o Kosher salt 1/2 tsp
o Ground black pepper 1/8 tsp
o Cheddar cheese shredded 1 cup
o Sour cream 1/4 cup

Steps of Preparation

o Place the cauliflower in a safe microwave plate and bake for 10 to 12 mins or till the pork is soft.
o Before microwave for the next thirty sec, add the cream cheese.
o Stir in the chicken, green salsa, pepper, salt, sour cream, cilantro& cheddar cheese.
o Bake for twenty mins inside an ovenproof baking dish in a preheated oven at 190 °, or you could have a 10-minute microwave on high. Serve warm.

33. Chicken crust pizza guilt-free

Total Time: 40 mins | Serving 8

Ingredients

o For Crust
o Fresh chicken breast 1.5 lbs.
o Minced garlic 2-3 cloves
o Blend Italian spice 1.5 tsp
o Shredded parmesan cheese 1/3 cup
o Shredded mozzarella cheese 1/3 cup
o Large egg 1
o For toppings
o Pasta sauce 3-4 tbsp
o Veggies
o Shredded mozzarella cheese 1/2 cup

o Shredded parmesan cheese 1/2 cup

Steps of Preparation

o Oven preheated to 400 ° c.

o Split the raw chicken into one "cubes & place it in small batches in a food processor to create some kind of handmade ground chicken.

o Place the raw ground chicken & the garlic, Italian spices, cheeses & egg in a bowl. Mix well.

o Line a baking sheet with a bakery release paper. Place the raw chicken combination ball on paper.

o Move out that much plastic wrap to covering the full pan or sheet and put it on top of the chicken combination ball. Push the chicken combination until it fills the pan or sheet.

o Pushed into two baking sheets for a lighter, crispier crust.

o Bake for almost 15 to 25 mins at 400 °, or till the crust becomes golden & to the desired crispness. Thicker crusts would be more about 20 to 25 mins & thin crusts take to cook in 10 to 15 mins.

o Take from the oven allow it to cool for around five mins.

o Distribute the sauce & top with the mozzarella. Apply the toppings & finish with the parmesan.

o Cook for 10 to 15 mins at 400 °, or till cheese seasoning has browned slightly.

o Cut, serve & enjoy this high protein meal that's free of guilt, low carb!

34. Asparagus stuffed chicken with parmesan

Servings: 3 | Total time: 30 min

Calories: 230 kcal | Proteins: 62 g | Carbohydrates: 10 g | Fat: 31 g

Ingredients

o Chicken Breasts 3

o Garlic paste 1 teaspoon

o Asparagus 12 Stalks

o Cream Cheese 1/2 cup

o Butter 1 tablespoon

o Olive Oil 1 teaspoon

o Marinara Sauce 3/4 cup

o shredded Mozzarella 1 cup

o Salt and Pepper

Steps of Preparation

o To start cooking the chicken, swirl the chicken (or split it in half without slicing it all
the way around. The chicken breast can open like a butterfly with one end already intact in the center). Remove the asparagus stalks and set it aside.

o Rub salt, some pepper, and garlic all across the chicken breasts (both in and out). Divide the cream cheese between all the chicken breasts and then spread to the inside. Now place four stalks of asparagus and afterward fold one side of that same breast over another, wrapping it in place with the help of a toothpick to ensure that it doesn't get open.

o Now preheat the oven, then set it to a broiler. Then Add butter and the olive oil to a hot saucepan and put the chicken breasts in it. Now took the breasts on either side for almost 6-7 minutes (the overall period would be 14-15 minutes based on the size of the breast) until the chicken will be almost cooked through.

o Now top each breast with almost 1/4 cup of marinara sauce and also top with shredded mozzarella. Put in the oven and bake

Chapter 3: Keto lunch recipes for women over 50

For women over 50 trying the keto diet, these simple keto lunch recipes are great and will help to get a balanced fat ketosis.

1. Keto avocado salad served with Blackened shrimp

Servings: 2 yields | Total time: 20 min

Calories: 420 kcal | Proteins: 49.5 g | Carbohydrates: 21 g | Fat: 18.5 g

Ingredients

o   One teaspoon crushed basil
o   One teaspoon black pepper
o   One teaspoon cayenne
o   Half kilogram peeled large shrimp
o   Two minced cloves of garlic
o   Two teaspoons paprika
o   One teaspoon dehydrated thyme
o   One teaspoon salt
o   Two bunches of Asparagus
o   One teaspoon of olive oil
o   Four cups lettuce leaves
o   One Avocado, diced
o   One fourth red onion, cut
o   One handful of basil leaves
o   One third cup greek yogurt
o   One teaspoon lemon pepper
o   One teaspoon lemon extract
o   Two tablespoons of water
o   Salt as required

Steps of preparation

o   In a narrow container, transfer shrimp and all other ingredients, and evenly coated it. Heat a big on medium flame and add some olive oil. Sauté the shrimp or prawns and the Asparagus, keep on turning seldom until they change color.
o   Now combine the lettuce leaves, the avocado, the onion slices, and the basil leaves in a glass bowl. Now add the shrimp or prawns and avocado. Add some dressing.
o   For the preparation of dressing, mix yogurt with the lemon pepper, the lemon juice, and the water and salt. Mix them well.

2. Keto Easy Egg Wrap lunch

Servings: 2 yields | Total time: 5 min

Calories: 411 kcal | Proteins: 25 g | Carbohydrates: 3 g | Fat: 31 g

Ingredients

o   Two Eggs
o   Boiled turkey
o   Mashed Avocado,
o   Crushed Cheese
o   Half teaspoon pepper,

- o Half teaspoon paprika,
- o Hummus
- o A pinch of salt
- o A pinch of cayenne pepper

Steps of preparation

- o Heat a shallow skillet over a medium heat. Use Butter or oil to grease.
- o Break one egg in a dish and blend well and with a fork.
- o Drop it in a hot skillet and tilt it to spread the egg into a wide circle at the bottom of the pan.
- o Let it simmer for 30 seconds.
- o Switch sides gently with a huge spatula and let it cook for the next 30 seconds.
- o Remove from heat and replicate the process for as number of eggs as you like to make.
- o Let the egg wraps cool down slightly (or completely), cover with the fillings as needed, wrap and serve it hot or cold.

3. Keto California Turkey and Bacon Lettuce Wraps with Basil-Mayo

Servings: 4 | Total time: 45 min

Calories: 303 kcal | Proteins: 11 g | Carbohydrates: 25 g | Fat: 20 g

Ingredients

- o One iceberg lettuce
- o Four slices of deli turkey
- o Four slices bacon
- o One diced avocado
- o One thinly diced tomato
- o Half cup mayonnaise
- o Six basil leaves
- o One teaspoon lemon extract
- o One chopped garlic clove
- o Salt as desired
- o Pepper as desired

Steps of preparation

- o To prepare Basil-Mayo, mix the ingredients in a food processor and process till smooth. n Optionally, mince both the basil and the garlic and mix them all together. This can be done in a couple of days ahead.
- o Place two wide leaves of lettuce on One slice of turkey and drench with Basil-Mayo. Put on a thin slice of turkey accompanied by bacon, including a couple of slices of avocado and the tomato. Season gently with salt and pepper, and then curl the bottom up as well as the sides in and roll it like a burrito. Cut halfway through, and then serve it cold.

4. Keto Lasagna Stuffed Portobellos

Servings: 4 yields | Total time: 25 min

Calories: 482 kcal | Proteins: 28 g | Carbohydrates: 6.5 g | Fat: 36 g

Ingredients

o Four mushrooms
o Four Italian sausage
o One milk mozzarella cheese
o One chopped parsley
o One cup of whole milk cheese
o One cup marinara sauce

Steps of preparation

o Clean the mushrooms. Remove the branches using a spoon.
o Take the sausage out and push the mixture into 4 patties. Force each patty into each of the mushroom cups, towards the edges and also up the sides of the Pattie.
o Now put 1/4 cup of the ricotta in each of the mushroom caps and then press the sides of it, creating a hole in the middle.
o Spoon 1/4 cup of sauce of marinara onto each mushroom on the highest point of the ricotta base.
o Sprinkle 1/4 cup of sliced mozzarella cheese on the top.
o Bake in a 375-degree F preheated oven for almost 40 minutes.
o Garnish it with parsley and serve when warm.

5. Rapid Keto Sushi

Servings: 3 yields | Total time: 25 min

Calories: 353 kcal | Proteins: 18.3 g | Carbohydrates: 5.7 g | Fat: 5.7 g

Ingredients

o One nori wrapper
o One cup of sliced cauliflower
o Half avocado
o One and a half oz Cream Cheese
o One fourth cup cucumber
o One tablespoon coconut oil
o One cup of soy sauce

Steps of preparation

o Split about half the head of the cauliflower into the florets and spin in the processor until the rice is appropriately smooth.
o Heat the coconut oil in a medium-high pan and introduce the cauliflower rice.
o Then Cook for almost 5-7 minutes till the rice is finely golden brown and cooked completely. Put it in a separate bowl.
o Slice the avocado, the cream cheese, and the cucumber into thinly sliced pieces and put them aside with the prepared cauliflower rice.
o Place a long sheet of plastic wrap on a clear, flat surface and place the nori wrapping above the plastic wrap.

- Cover the cauliflower rice over all the nori wrapping as thinly or as dense as you want in an even coating. Leave some room around the corners and edges.
- For some keto sushi rice, apply the first coating of the avocado on the rice adjacent to you. Next, add a thin layer of some cream cheese straight to the avocado, and finally, add a layer of cucumber.
- For keto sushi cucumber, firs raise the plastic wrap on the side by using your palms to mask the ingredients.
- Steadily stretch the plastic wrap and the nori wraps over the avocado, the cucumber, and the cream cheese before you cover the whole.
- Using a sharp knife, split the sushi into eight parts. First, Begin in the center so that the rice is not pulled out along with the weight of the knife.

6. Chicken Piccata keto Meatballs

Serving: 3 | Total: Time 30 min

Calories: 323 kcal, Fat:21g, Net Carbs:2g Protein:26g

Ingredients

- Ground chicken 1 lb.
- Almond flour 1/3 cup
- Egg 1
- Kosher salt 1/2 tsp
- Ground black pepper 1/4 tsp
- Garlic powder 1/4 tsp
- Lemon zest 1/2 tsp
- Fresh chopped parsley 1 tsp
- Olive oil 2 tbsp

For the sauce:

- Dry white wine 1/2 cup
- Lemon juice 2 tbsp
- Drained & chopped capers 2 tbsp
- Lemon zest 1/4 tsp
- Butter 1/4 cup

Steps of Preparation

- In a med bowl, mix the ground meat, almond meal/flour, egg, pepper, salt, powder of garlic, zest of the lemon as well as parsley together & stir thoroughly. Form into fifteen meatballs. Heat the oil of olive in a non-stick skillet & cook the meatballs till they become golden brown & fried through.
- In the same skillet as the meatballs were cooked, add the white wine & bring to a simmer, having to scrape all the meatballs off the skillet & into the white wine. Apply the juice of lemon & capers and reduce by around half (2 to 3 mins). Turn off the heat & stir in the zest of lemon & butter till melted as well as smooth. sprinkle with salt to taste

7. Keto Chicken Alfredo Spaghetti Squash

Servings: 4| Total Time: 20 mins

Calories: 327 kcal |Fat:25g | Net Carbs:14g| Protein:12g

Ingredients

- 2 tbsp butter
- Minced Garlic 2 tsp
- Sage 1 tsp
- Flour 2tbsp
- Chicken broth 1 cup
- Half cream 1/2 cup
- Cubed cream cheese 4 oz
- Shredded parmesan cheese ½ cup
- Cooked & shredded chicken 1/2 cup
- Cooked spaghetti squash 2 1/2 cups
- Pepper, salt & parsley

Steps of Preparation

- Melt the butter over med-heat in a pan.
- Add the sage & garlic, then cook for around a min.
- Mix in the flour/meal & cook, constantly mixing for around a minute.
- Mix a half & half in a chicken broth.
- Mix in the parmesan cheese & cream cheese till smooth.
- Add the vegetable squash, cooked and shredded chicken, & cook till fully heated.
- Taste the alfredo vegetable squash with chicken, then top with pepper, salt & parsley.

8. Keto Paleo lunch Spice Chicken Skewers

Serving 2| Total Time: 2 hours

Calories: 198 |Fat:5g | Net Carbs |1g Protein:35g

Ingredients

- Boneless & skinless chicken tenders 2 lb.
- Granulated erythritol sweetener 2 tbsp
- 5 spice powder 2 tbsp
- Rice wine vinegar unsweetened 1 tbsp
- Avocado oil 1 tbsp
- Sesame oil 1 tsp
- Gluten-free soy sauce 1 tbsp
- Skewers red bell pepper pieces 1 cup
- Skewers 12

Steps of Preparation

- Cut the chicken finely into pieces just around two inches long onto the diagonal.
- In a med bowl, mix the sweetener, five powder spice, rice wine vinegar, oil of avocado, oil of sesame, soy sauce & cayenne pepper & stir.
- Season & adjust sweetness/saltiness according to your preference.

- Apply the pieces of chicken, then mix well to coat.
- Marinate a chicken for one hr. or more, & up to twenty-four hrs.
- Heat the grill.
- Thread pieces of chicken & red bell pepper onto the skewers.
- Grill each side for 2 -3 mins or once the chicken is cooked through.
- When desired, garnish with lime slices & cilantro (fresh).

9. Keto Asian pork ribs

| Serving 4 | Total Time 1 hr.

Calories: 505 |Fat: 44g |Net Carbs: 1g |Protein: 25g

Ingredients

- Chopped pork spareribs into individual ribs 2 lb.
- Fresh diced ginger 1 tbsp
- Diced green onions 2 tbsp
- Szechuan peppercorns ½ tbsp
- 2-star anise
- Diced garlic cloves 3
- Gluten-free tamari sauce or coconut amino 2 tbsp
- Avocado oil 2 tbsp
- Salt & pepper to taste

Steps of Preparation

- To a big pot of boiling water, add flour, Szechuan peppercorns, star anise, & ribs. Bring to boil, then cook till the meat is soft, for 45 mins. Skim away any shaping foam.
- Drain from the pot & remove ribs. Remove the star anise & peppercorns.
- Apply the avocado oil to the frying pan, then add the ginger and garlic. Put in ribs & cook on the medium-high fire. Add the coconut amino or tamari sauce, then season, to taste, with pepper and salt.
- Stir-fry ribs over high heat until fully covered and browned with the sauce.

10. Keto slow cooker pork's rib (Asian)

Servings: 2 | Total Time:3hrs. 20 mins

Calories: 482 |Fat: 38g| Net Carbs: 4g |Protein: 25g

Ingredients

- Baby back pork ribs 450g
- Sliced medium onion 1/2
- Garlic paste 1 tbsp
- Ginger paste 1 tbsp
- Chicken broth 1&1/2 c
- Gluten-free tamari sauce or coconut amino 2 tbsp
- Chinese five-spice seasoning ½ tsp
- Sliced green onions 2

Steps of Preparation

o Place the pork ribs rack inside the slow cooker. The rack may need to be halved to fit.

o Include the onions, paste for garlic, paste for the ginger, and broth for the meat. If the ribs are not completely coated, add up a little bit of broth until covered.

o Cover & cook for three hours at low flame.

o To keep warm, remove ribs & wrap in foil. Place this apart.

o Shift the onions & products from the slow cooker into the stove to a clean pan. Using a hand blender, blitz well (or use a food processor to blitz and move to the stove in the pan) and apply the Chinese 5-spice & tamari. Reduce the paste to dense and jammy, over a relatively high flame.

o Taste the marinade and add in a bit of erythritol if you think it will improve from a little more sugar.

o Brush over the warm ribs with this marinade & garnish with onions.

11. Keto baked ribs recipe

Serving 2 | Total Time: 3hrs. 5 mins

Calories 580 | Fat: 51g | Net Carbs: 5g | Protein: 25g

Ingredients

o Baby back ribs 1 lb.

o Applesauce 2 tbsp

o Gluten-free tamari sauce or coconut amino 2 tbsp

o Olive oil 2 tbsp

o Fresh ginger 1 tbsp

o Garlic cloves 2

o Salt & pepper

Steps of Preparation

o Preheat the oven to 275 F— change it to the minimum temperature if your oven does not go down to this point.

o Season with salt & pepper over ribs & cover securely with foil. Put the product onto a baking dish and bake in the oven for three hours at low temp.

o Mix olive oil, applesauce, tamari sauce, ginger, and garlic in a blender until it creates a purée.

o Take the ribs out from the oven after three hours, then adjust the heat in the oven up to 450 F (230 C) or just as high as the oven can go.

o With care, open the foil so the ribs can rest on top of the foil. Coat the ribs well with the marinade, by using a brush. Put the ribs in the oven and bake for 5-10 mins till it becomes sticky with marinade.

12. Keto fried pork tenderloin

Serving 2 | Total Time: 20 mins

Calories: 389 Kcal | Fat: 23g |Net Carbs: 0g |Protein: 47g

Ingredients

o Pork tenderloin 1 lb.
o Salt & pepper>> to taste
o Avocado or coconut oil 2 tbsp

Steps of Preparation

o Break the pork tenderloin into two-three pieces to fit more conveniently into your frying pan.
o Apply the oil to the frying pan & fry the pork tenderloin first on one side, using tongs. Using tongs, flip the pork tenderloin until that side is fried, then cook the other side until both sides are browned.
o Continue to turn the pork every several minutes till the meat thermometer displays just below 145F (63C), internal temperature. Since you remove it from the frying pan, the pork will begin to cook a little.
o Let the pork rest for a couple of minutes then slice with a knife into one-inch-thick slices.

13. Cauliflower Grits with shrimps and Arugula

Servings: 4 yields | Total time: 30 min

Calories: 122 kcal | Proteins: 16 g | Carbohydrates: 3 g | Fat: 5 g

Ingredients

o One-pound peeled shrimp
o One tablespoon bell pepper crushed
o Two teaspoons garlic paste
o Half teaspoon cayenne pepper
o One tablespoon olive oil
o Salt and freshly ground black pepper
o One tablespoon butter
o Four cups riced cauliflower
o One cup milk
o Half cup crumbled goat cheese
o Salt and freshly ground black pepper
o One tablespoon olive oil
o Three diced garlic cloves
o Four cups arugula
o Salt and black pepper as desired

Steps of preparation

o Put the shrimp in a big plastic zip bag. In a medium container, mix the paprika with some garlic powder and the cayenne. Put the mixture to the shrimp bag and toss well until the spices are covered. Refrigerate when you're preparing the grits.

- Melt the butter in a medium pot over medium heat. Include the cauliflower rice and cook till some moisture is produced, that is 2 to 3 minutes.
- Mix in half milk and bring to boil. Allow it to boil, keep stirring regularly, until some milk is absorbed by the cauliflower for; it will happen in 6 to 8 minutes.
- Incorporate the leftover milk and boil until the mixture is dense and smooth, cook for 10 minutes. Mix with goat cheese and then season it with some salt and pepper. Keep it warm.

14. Keto Chipotle Pork Wraps

Servings: 2 yields | Total time: 15 min

Calories: 292 kcal | Proteins: 14 g | Carbohydrates: 37 g | Fat: 0 g

Ingredients

- Half Avocado
- Two tablespoons Mayonnaise
- One lime juice extract
- One clove of garlic minced
- Salt and pepper as required
- Water
- One Head Iceberg Lettuce
- Two cups Pork
- One Avocado

Steps of preparation

- Mash the avocado and sweep in the mayonnaise, garlic, lime juice, and some salt and pepper. If the aioli wants to be thin, then apply a little bit of water so that it can be quickly drizzled.
- Place the pork in the lettuce cups, cover with the sliced avocado, and drizzle it with the aioli and cover with cilantro and some lime.

15. Keto Italian Chicken Meal Prep Bowls

Servings: 2 yields | Total time: 15 min

Calories: 292 kcal | Proteins: 14 g | Carbohydrates: 37 g | Fat: 0 g

Ingredients

- One teaspoon salt
- half t teaspoon pepper
- Two teaspoon basil
- Two teaspoon marjoram
- Two teaspoon rosemary
- Two teaspoon thyme
- Two teaspoons paprika
- Two pounds boneless skinless chicken breasts cut into bite-sized pieces
- One and a half cup broccoli florets
- One small red chopped onion
- One cup tomato
- One medium zucchini chopped
- Two teaspoons minced garlic

- Two Tablespoon olive oil
- Two cups cooked rice

Steps of preparation

- Preheat the oven to 450F. Then Line the baking sheet of aluminum foil and put it aside.
- In a small container, add some salt, some pepper, marjoram, some rosemary, basil, thyme, and paprika.
- Put chicken and vegetables in the baking bowl. Spray all the seasoning and garlic equally over all the chicken as well as the vegetables. Then Drizzle with some olive oil.
- Now Bake for almost 15-20 minutes unless the chicken is properly cooked and vegetables are finely crispy.
- Broil the brown chicken for 1-2 minutes.
- Put 1/2 or 1 cup of the cooked rice of your preference in four different preparation containers.
- Segregate chicken and vegetables equally all over the rice.
- Cover them, and them keep in the refrigerator for 3-5 days, or you can serve them for dinner.

16. Cheeseburger Lettuce Wraps

Servings: 1 | Total time: 15 min

Calories: 556 kcal | Proteins: 33.6 g | Carbohydrates: 8.2 g | Fat: 42 g

Ingredients

- Two pounds minced beef
- Half teaspoon salts
- One teaspoon black pepper
- One teaspoon oregano
- Six slices of American cheese
- Two heads iceberg
- Two tomatoes diced
- One fourth cup light mayo
- Three tablespoons ketchup
- One Tablespoon relish
- salt and pepper as required

Steps of preparation

- First, heat the grill or the skillet over medium temperature.
- In a large container, add some ground beef, some seasoned salt, and pepper, and some oregano.
- Now Divide the mixture into six parts and then curl each of them into a ball. Squeeze each ball down to create a patty.
- Put the patties on the grill or the pan and then cook for almost 4 minutes from either direction or till cooked to desired taste. (when using a grill, just prepare 3 min at a time to avoid congestion).

- Put a piece of cheese on top of the grilled burgers. Put each cheeseburger on a broad lettuce leaf. Cover with spreading and one slice of tomato, some red onion, and whatever you want. Wrap the lettuce over the top then eat. Savor it!
- In a little pan, add all the components of the spread. Put it in the fridge before available for usage.

17. Classic Stuffed Peppers

Servings: 6 | Total time: 1 hour 20 min

Calories: 376 kcal | Proteins: 16 g | Carbohydrates: 52 g | Fat: 12 g

Ingredients

- Six bell peppers
- One-pound ground beef
- One minced onion
- Two minced garlic cloves
- Three fourth cup boiled rice
- One teaspoon paprika
- Half teaspoon oregano
- Half teaspoon mustard powder
- Half cup parsley
- Salt and black pepper
- Half cup Jack cheese

Steps of preparation

- Preheat to 375 ° F in the oven. Apply the marinara sauce to the center of a medium-sized skillet.

- Prune the base within each pepper a bit, so it lies flat. Break off the tops of each pepper and then detach the ribs and the seeds and then discard them.
- In a medium dish, combine beef with onion, paprika, oregano, garlic, rice, mustard pepper, and some parsley and salt
- Load the mixture of meat into each of the peppers, filling up to the top. Shift the peppers to the heated skillet and put them on the upper edge of the sauce.
- Garnish with one and a half teaspoons of cheese. Bake until the peppers are juicy, and the beef is thoroughly cooked for 25 to 30 minutes. Serve straight away with some scoop of sauce.

18. Chicken Lemon herb Mediterranean salad

Servings: 1 | Total time: 15 min

Calories: 336 kcal | Proteins: 24 g | Carbohydrates: 13 g | Fat: 21 g

Ingredients

- Two tablespoons olive oil
- One lemon juice extract
- Two tablespoons of water
- Two tablespoons of vinegar
- Two tablespoons of parsley

- Two teaspoons basil
- Two teaspoons of minced garlic
- Two teaspoons of oregano
- One teaspoon of salt
- One pepper
- One-pound boneless chicken thigh fillets
- Four cups Romaine lettuce leaves
- One diced cucumber
- Two tomatoes cubed
- One red onion cubed
- One diced avocado
- One-third cup rutted Kalamata olives

Steps of preparation

- In a big container, mix together all the marinade components. Add half of the marinade to a big, shallow pan. Refrigerate the leftover marinade for further use as a topping.
- In a bowl, add chicken to some marinade and marinate the chicken for 15-30 minutes (and for up to 2 hours in the fridge if time allows). When waiting for the chicken to marinate, arrange all the components of the salad, and combine in a big bowl of salad.
- When chicken is prepared, warm 1 tablespoon of olive oil inside a grill pan or grill above medium-high heat. Barbecue chicken from both sides until golden brown and cooked completely.

- Keep chicken to settle for 5 min; cut and place over the salad. Drizzle with the leftover unchanged dressing. End up serving with a lemon slice.

19. Keto BLT stuffed chicken salad avocados

Servings: 1 | Total time: 30 min

Calories: 267 kcal | Proteins: 14 g | Carbohydrates: 13.6 g | Fat: 17 g

Ingredients

- Twelve slices of turkey bacon
- One and a half cups of shredded rotisserie chicken
- Two tomatoes
- One and a half cups of cottage cheese
- One cup of finely chopped lettuce
- Three avocados

Steps of preparation

- Preheat the oven to the temperature of 400 degrees F.
- Place Twelve slices of the turkey bacon on a parchment lining the baking dish
- Bake for almost 10 minutes, then rotate, and bake for the next five minutes, then scatter the bacon over a few sheets of some paper towels to it cool off.
- In the meantime, quarter the tomatoes, scrape out all the pulp and the seeds with

the help of fingertips, and break into tiny bits.

o Cut the Romaine into little bits

o In a big bowl, add meat, some cottage cheese, some romaine, some berries, turkey bacon, and combine together.

o Sprinkle with salt and pepper as desired.

o Half the avocados cut the pits and then season gently with some salt and pepper.

o Scoop 1/6 (roughly) of the chicken salad inside each avocado. Not a massive amount is going to fit into the hole produced by the seed, so you're going to add a good amount on upper edge of the avocado.

20. Cheesy taco skillet

Servings: 6 yields | Total time: 30 min

Calories: 241 kcal | Proteins: 30 g | Carbohydrates: 9 g | Fat: 20 g

Ingredients

o One-pound ground beef

o One diced large yellow onion

o Two diced bell peppers

o One diced tomato

o One shredded large zucchini

o taco seasoning

o Three cups pf baby kale

o One and a half cup of shredded cheddar cheese

Steps of preparation

o In a wide pan, gently cook ground beef and also well crumble.

o Drain the waste of fat.

o Include the onions and the peppers and cook till golden.

o Add some canned tomatoes, some taco seasoning, as well as any water required for taco seasoning to uniformly cover the mixture (up to 1 tablespoon – the tomato liquid may benefit)

o Apply the greens and make it absolutely wilt.

o Mix it finely.

21. Cauliflower Cheesy Breadsticks

Servings: 8 | Total time: 43 min

Calories: 102 kcal | Proteins: 7.1 g | Carbohydrates: 1.1 g | Fat: 7.7 g

Ingredients

o Four cups of diced cauliflower

o Four eggs

o Two cups of mozzarella

o Three teaspoon oregano

o Four minced cloves of garlic

o Salt and pepper as desired

o One cup of mozzarella cheese

Steps of preparation

- Start by Preheating the oven to a temperature of 425 ° F. Arrange Two pizza plates or a broad baking sheet with parchment paper on them.
- Try to make sure the florets of cauliflower are finely cut. Apply the florets to the processor and spin.
- In a microwaveable jar, put the cauliflower then cover it with a lid. Microwave it for a time of 10-minutes. Only let cauliflower cool until there was no steam rising from it anymore. Put in a wide bowl the microwave cauliflower and transfer oregano, 2 cups mozzarella, salt, garlic, and pepper to the whites. Mix in everything.
- Segregate the mixture into two and put each half on the ready baking sheets and form the breadsticks either into a pizza crust or in a rectangular shape.
- Bake the crust for around 25 minutes (no covering yet) till it is soft and brown. Don't be scared; the crust isn't soggy. Sprinkle with the leftover mozzarella cheese once golden and bring it oven and bake for the next five min just until the cheese is melted.
- Start Slicing and serving.

22. Loaded cauliflower

Servings: 4 | Total time: 15 min

Calories: 298 kcal | Proteins: 7.4 g | Carbohydrates: 1.1 g | Fat: 24.6 g

Ingredients

- One-pound cauliflower
- Four ounces of sour cream
- One cup of grated cheddar cheese
- Two slices of bacon
- Two tablespoons of chives
- Three tablespoons of butter
- One fourth teaspoon of garlic paste
- Salt and pepper as required

Steps of preparation

- Slice the cauliflower into the form of florets and transfer them to a suitable bowl within microwave. Add almost 2 teaspoons of water and soak with film that sticks. Microwave for another 5-8 minutes, before fully cooked and soft, based on the microwave. Dump the extra water and allow for a couple of seconds to stay uncovered. (Alternately, the traditional method, boil the cauliflower. Upon boiling, you can need to drain a little extra water out from inside the cauliflower.
- In a food processor, add the cauliflower and process it until soft. Introduce the butter, and sour cream, and garlic powder, then process to the texture of mashed potatoes. Remove the mashed

cauliflower to a pot and mix much of the chives, leaving any later to apply to the end. add the rest of the sharp cheddar cheese and combine through hand. Sprinkle some salt and pepper as desired.

o Cover the filled cauliflower with the remainder cheese, leftover chives, and some bacon. To melt the cheese, place it in the microwave or place cauliflower for another few minutes under the broiler.

23. Keto Grilled tuna salad

Servings: 2 | Total time: 1 hour

Calories: 975 kcal | Proteins: 53 g | Carbohydrates: 9 g | Fat: 79 g

Ingredients

o Two large egg
o Eight ounces of asparagus
o One tablespoon of olive oil
o Eight ounces of fresh tuna
o Four ounces of spring mix
o Four ounces of cherry tomatoes
o Half red onion
o Two tablespoons of chopped walnuts
o Half cup of mayonnaise
o Two tablespoons of water
o Two teaspoons of garlic paste
o Salt and pepper were required

Steps for preparation

o Gather all of the things for preparation.

o Add the water, the garlic powder, mayonnaise, and salt, and the pepper together in a bowl to create the dressing. Mix until well blended and set it aside.

o Boil the eggs for 8-10 minutes or so. Peel and break in half until cooled.

o Clean and split the asparagus onto similar lengths. In a pan, cook the asparagus.

o Pour the olive oil between both sides of the tuna in the same manner and fry it on both sides for 3-5 minutes. To taste, sprinkle the tuna with the salt and the pepper.

o Put the leafy greens, the cherry tomatoes (sliced in half), onion, and the eggs on a tray.

o Slice into pieces of the cooked tuna and put it on top. On the top of the salad, pour the dressing sauce and scatter the sliced walnuts on top of that.

24. Creamy ketogenic taco soup

Servings: 4 | Total time: 35 min

Calories: 345 kcal | Proteins: 21 g | Carbohydrates: 5 g | Fat: 27 g

Ingredients

o Sixteen ounces of ground beef
o One tablespoon of olive oil
o One medium diced onion
o Three minced cloves of garlic

- One diced green bell pepper
- Ten ounces of canned tomatoes
- One cup of heavy cream
- Two tablespoons of taco seasoning
- Salt and pepper as required
- Two cups of beef broth
- One medium cubed avocado
- Four tablespoons of sour cream
- Four tablespoons of cilantro

Steps of preparation

- Gather all of the supplies. Dice the bell pepper and the onion long in advance.
- Add the olive oil, onion, and ground beef and garlic, to a small saucepan over medium heat. Sprinkle salt and pepper, season.
- Cook it until golden brown beef and transparent onion.
- Add some bell pepper, heavy cream, sliced tomatoes with green chili, and taco seasoning until the beef is golden brown.
- Simmer together properly to guarantee that all of the products contain the spices and seasoning.
- Transfer the water to the beef and then get the soup to a simmer. Decrease the heat to low and simmer for almost 10-15 minutes or until liquid is decreased, and soup is prepared according to the desired

taste. If needed, try and add salt and pepper.
- Add the sour cream and the cilantro avocado to the portions and garnish. Add a squeeze of lime juice, too.

25. Keto fish cakes with dipping sauce

Servings: 6 | Total time: 15 min

Calories: 69 kcal | Proteins: 53 g | Carbohydrates: 2.7 g | Fat: 6.5 g

Ingredients

- One-pound raw white boneless fish
- One by four cup of cilantro
- Salt as required
- Chili flakes as required
- Two garlic cloves
- Two tablespoons of coconut oil
- Two ripe avocados
- One lemon juice extract
- Two tablespoons of water

Steps of preparation

- Put the fish, vegetables, garlic (if used), spice, chili, and fish in a processor. Blitz before everything is equally mixed.
- Apply the coconut oil to a wide frying pan over medium-high heat and stir the pan.
- Oil the hands and roll in Six patties of the fish combination.

- To the hot frying pan and add the cakes. Cook till lightly browned and fried thru, on both sides.
- While the fish cakes are frying, in a blender, incorporate all the dipping sauce components (starting with lemon juice) and mix thoroughly until it becomes fluffy. Taste the mixture and apply, if necessary, other lemon juice or salt.
- Serve hot with the dipping sauce when the fish cakes become baked.

26. Ketogenic Paleo Meat Ball for lunch

Servings: 3 | Total time: 30 min

Calories: 475 kcal | Proteins: 61.3 g | Carbohydrates: 5.6 g | Fat: 21.7 g

Ingredients

- One and a half pounds of ground beef
- Two tablespoons ghee
- One tablespoon apple cider vinegar
- Half teaspoon of pepper
- One teaspoon of salt
- Yellow minced onion
- Two minced garlic cloved
- One fourth cup of chopped rosemary

Steps of preparation

- Start by Preheating the oven to the temperature of 350 degrees ° C.

- Put all the meatballs supplies in a bowl and mix, and when well mixed, use the hands to combine it together.
- Line a parchment paper on baking tray and fold the mixture into tiny balls, utilizing approximately a tablespoon of mix per meatball.
- Now meatballs are wrapped and placed on the parchment. Bake for almost 20 minutes or until baked completely.
- Serve hot or allow it to cool and seal in the refrigerator in an airtight jar.

27. Ketogenic Mexican Shredded beef

Servings: 20 | Total time: 3-hour 20 min

Calories: 323 kcal | Proteins: 53 g | Carbohydrates: 7.3 g | Fat: 12.9 g

Ingredients

- Three and a half pounds beef short ribs
- Two teaspoons turmeric powder
- One teaspoon salt
- Half teaspoon peppers
- Two teaspoons cumin powder
- Two teaspoons coriander powder
- Half cup waters
- One cup cilantro chopped

Steps of preparation

- Combine the dried ingredients in a shallow pan.

- For a slow cooker, introduce short ribs and gently brush each bit in the seasoning mix.
- Scatter over the ribs with cilantro stems and additional garlic. Apply water carefully without scrubbing the spices off.
- On low heat, cook for 6-7 hours, or until it falls apart. After 6 hours, inspect the beef and cook further when it's not soft enough.
- Drain the cooking liquid in a medium pan if necessary and decrease it over a moderate flame for 15 minutes.
- Transfer the liquid back into another crockpot. Take off the steak and cut the beef utilizing two forks.
- Serve warm with guacamole, taco-like silverbeet leaves, corn, cucumbers, organic cilantro, and green beans.

28. Keto low carb pork & cashew stir fry

Total Time: 10 mins | Servings: 2 |

Calories: 403 kcal | Fat: 27g |Net Carbs: 12g | Protein: 28g

Ingredients

- Avocado oil 2 tbsp
- Shredded pork ½ lb.
- Sliced green bell pepper ½
- Sliced red bell pepper ½
- Sliced medium onion 1/4
- Cashews 1/3 c
- Fresh grated ginger 1 tbsp
- Minced cloves of garlic 3
- Chinese chili oil 1 tsp
- Sesame oil 1 tbsp
- Gluten-free tamari sauce or coconut amino 2 tbsp
- Salt>> to taste

Steps of Preparation

- Put avocado oil in a frying saucepan & cook the pork (if uncooked).
- Next, add onions, pepper & cashews, all sliced.
- Sauté until completely cooked pork. Then mix in ginger, garlic, tamari sauce, chili oil, sesame oil & salt to your taste.

29. Keto pork stuffed with sausages & cauliflower rice

Total Time: 30 mins | Serving 4
Calories: kcal 473 | Fat: 24g | Net Carbs: 3g |Protein: 57g

Ingredients

- Avocado oil 4 tbsp
- Minced garlic cloves 2
- Small cauliflower cut into small rice-like particles ¼
- Chopped onion 1 tbsp
- Chopped red bell pepper 1 tbsp
- Chopped sausage ½
- Green peas 1 tbsp
- Pork tenderloin 1&1/2 lb.

o Salt & pepper>> to taste

Steps of Preparation

o Preheat the oven before 400 F (200 C).

o Pour 2 Tsp of avocado oil over moderate temp in a wide skillet, then add garlic & onion. Cook them, till the onion is transparent, for a few minutes.

o Stir in the cauliflower, sausage, red pepper & roast for ten minutes. Season with salt & pepper.

o Slice the pork tenderloin to open it lengthwise but don't cut through. Using a meat pounder, pound meat if you've it.

o Cover with rice mixture halfway over the tenderloin. Wrap meat up & use twine to bind it together. (use cocktail sticks to protect the pork If you don't have twine.)

o In a separate frying pan, melt two tbsp of avocado oil. Crisp up the pork tenderloin gently on either side for a few minutes until it is brown.

o Place your filled pork tenderloin upon the baking tray and let them steam for at least thirty minutes uncovered. If you have got a meat thermometer, this should display 145 F.

o Let the meat sit for ten minutes before the strings are cut and sliced.

30. Keto pork tenderloin stuffed with cabbage

Total Time: 40 mins | Serving: 4

Calories: 207 kcal | Fat: 12g | Net Carbs: 2g | Protein: 24g

Ingredients

o Avocado oil 2 tbsp
o Diced onion ¼
o Diced cabbage 1 c
o Minced garlic cloves 2
o Salt & pepper>> to taste
o Pork tenderloin 1 lb.

Steps of Preparation

o Preheat the oven before 400 F (200 C).

o Apply the avocado oil over medium heat to a frying pan and sauté the cabbage, onions, garlic till cabbage is soft. Season to taste, with salt & black pepper.

o Lengthwise slit the tenderloin but do not cut into it all the way completely. Using it to hammer the pork tenderloin to a big flat slice (approx. ½-inch-thick), if you have got a meat pounder.

o Place the flat tenderloin over a cutting board & put the fried cabbage in the center.

o Roll up and cover the tenderloin with twine or use cocktail sticks to roast.

- Place it on a baking dish and take 40 mins. Testing the pork achieves an inner temp of 145 F.

31. Keto marinated pork tenderloin

Total Time: 20 mins | Serving 4

Calories: 258 kcal | Fat: 19g | Net Carbs: 1g | Protein: 24g

Ingredients

- Cut into 2 long pieces of pork tenderloin 1lb.
- Olive oil ¼ c
- Greek seasoning 2 tbsp
- Red wine vinegar 1 tbsp
- Lemon juice 1 tbsp
- Salt & pepper

for Greek Seasoning:

- Garlic powder 1 tsp
- Dried oregano 1tsp
- Dried basil 1tsp
- Dried rosemary ½ tsp
- Dried thyme ½ tsp
- Dried dill ½ tsp
- Cinnamon ½ tsp
- Parsley ½ tsp
- Marjoram ½ tsp

Steps of Preparation

- Mix the olive oil, vinegar, lemon juice & seasoning in a big zip lock container.
- Put the 2 pieces of pork tenderloin in the container and marinate in the fridge overnight.
- Place the pork over medium heat in a frying pan. Place the pork with one side and roast. Then by using tongs, turn the pork into a good browning on every side.
- Continue to turn the pork till the inner temp reaches 145 F/63 C (control using a meat thermometer).

32. Keto herbs pork tenderloin

Total Time: 20 mins | Serving 2

Total Time: kcal: 627 | Fat: 49g | Net Carbs: 4g | Protein: 44g

Ingredients

- Pine nut 2 tbsp
- Chopped garlic cloves 3
- Fresh basil leaves 1 c
- Fresh parsley ½ c + 2 tbsp
- Nutritional yeast 2 tbsp
- Olive oil 5 tbsp
- Juice of 1 lemon
- salt to taste

For the pork

- Pork tenderloin 14 oz
- Salt & ground black pepper
- Olive oil 1 tbsp
- Reserved herbs paste 3 tbsp

Steps of Preparation

o Begin by toasting pine nuts in a heavy, dry skillet to create the herb paste. Take out the crispy pine nuts and apply the garlic, basil, nutritional yeast flakes, fresh parsley, and olive oil to a mini food processor. Combine to make a perfect paste, scraping many times across the sides of the container. Season with salt & lemon juice to taste. Place on the side.

o Preheat oven to 410 ° F (210 ° C) for pork.

o Season the pork tenderloin on both sides with salt and freshly ground black pepper. In a non-stick pan, heat the olive oil & brown the tenderloin at both sides. Remove from heat and let it cool down a little bit. Using a palette knife or thin silicone spatula until cool enough to treat, then spread the stored herb paste over the pork tenderloin on both sides. Put tenderloin with a well-equipped cover in a casserole dish & cook in the oven for 12-15 mins or till cooked to your taste.

o Remove from oven and enable it to cool before sliced and served. Serve with some extra herbs paste if needed.

33. Keto basil pork Fettucine

Total Time: 15 mins | Servings: 3

Calories: 231 | Fat: 16g | Net Carbs: 5g |Protein: 16g

Ingredients

o 5 packs of fettuccine shirataki noodles of 3 oz

o coconut oil 2 tbsp

o Pork tenderloin ½ lb.

o salt & pepper>> to taste

o Sliced leek 1

o Chopped garlic cloves 2

o coconut cream 4 tbsp

o Fresh chopped basil leaves ¼ c

o Dash of chicken broth

Steps of Preparation

o To 400 F, preheat the oven.

o Rinse under cool, flowing water the shirataki noodles, and hold warm in a pot of softly simmering water upon a burner.

o Heat 1 tbsp of coconut oil in a wide saucepan and brown both sides of the pork tenderloin. Take the pork off the skillet & season with salt & black pepper. Shift the pork to a baking tray and put over it in the oven for ten min. Remove, and then let rest.

o Meanwhile, heat in the same pan the remaining coconut oil used for the pork & cook the leeks & garlic over medium heat until soft. For keeping the mixture moist,

apply a splash of chicken broth. Apply
the coconut cream & basil once wet.

o Drain the hot noodles and put them in a
bowl. Spoon over sauce with leek. Cut the
pork & put it on top of the sauce.

o

Chapter 4: Keto Dinner Recipes for Women above 50

These are some keto dinner recipes for women above 50. These recipes are simple, easy, and fulfill all the requirements of the body by keeping you healthy and fit.

1. Creamy Tuscan garlic chicken

Servings: 6 | Total time: 25 min

Calories: 368 kcal | Proteins: 30 g | Carbohydrates: 7 g | Fat: 25 g

Ingredients

o One and a half pounds of boneless chicken breasts

o Two Tablespoons of olive oil

o One cup cream

o Half cup of chicken broth

o One teaspoon of garlic powder

o One teaspoon of italian seasoning

o Half cup of parmesan cheese

o One cup spinach chopped

o Half cup tomatoes dried

Steps of preparation

o Put olive oil in a wide skillet and cook chicken on medium-high heat for 3-5 minutes per side or until golden around each side and cook until the middle is no longer pink. Remove the chicken then put that aside on a tray.

o Transfer some chicken broth, heavy cream, Italian seasoning, garlic powder, and parmesan cheese. Mix over medium-high heat unless it begins to thicken. Include the spinach and the sundried tomatoes and boil before the spinach starts wilting. Add the chicken to the skillet and, if needed, pour over pasta.

o Serve with a lemon slice.

2. Avocado Greek salad

Servings: 4 | Total time: 15 min

Calories: 305 kcal | Proteins: 10 g | Carbohydrates: 12 g | Fat: 27 g

Ingredients

o One by four cup olive oil

o Two tablespoons vinegar

o One teaspoon garlic paste

o Two teaspoons dried oregano

o One fourth teaspoon salt

o One large sliced cucumber

o Four wedge cut tomatoes

o One green pepper sliced

o Half sliced red onion

o 200 g cubed creamy feta cheese

o Half cup olives

o One large diced avocado

Steps of preparation

o Mix together the spices of the dressing in the jar.

o In a bowl, combine all the ingredients of the salad. Toss the dressing. Season with some salt only if required (depending about how salty your feta cheese is). Sprinkle on additional oregano to use. Start serving with chicken, lamb, beef, fish; the choices are infinite!

3. Keto Eggs and Zoodles

Servings: 2 | Total time: 25 min

Calories: 633 kcal | Proteins: 20 g | Carbohydrates: 27 g | Fat: 53 g

Ingredients

o Nonstick spray

o Three zucchinis

o Two tablespoons olive oil

o A pinch of Kosher salt and black pepper

o Four large eggs

o Red-pepper flakes

o Basil

o Two thinly sliced avocados

Steps of preparation

o Preheat oven to 350 ° degrees F. Lightly oil a nonstick spray baking sheet.

o In a wide pan, mix the zucchini noodles with the olive oil. Season to taste with the salt and the pepper. Divide into Four even parts, move to the baking tray, and build a nest shape.

o steadily crack the egg in the center of each nest. Bake until eggs are ready, for 9 to 11 minutes. Season to taste with salt and pepper, garnish with red pepper flakes and basil. Serve with the slices of avocado.

4. Cheese and the Cauliflower 'Breadsticks

Servings: 4 | Total time: 20 min

Calories: 200 kcal | Proteins: 12 g | Carbohydrates: 9 g | Fat: 14 g

Ingredients

o One head cauliflower

o Two garlic cloves

o One third cup mozzarella cheese

o One third cup Parmesan cheese

o Two eggs

o One egg white

o One tablespoon thyme

o One tablespoon rosemary chopped

o A pinch of Kosher salt and black pepper

o Two tablespoons of olive oil

Steps of preparation

- Begin by preheating the oven to a temperature of 425 ° F. Cover a baking sheet of parchment paper.
- In a food processor bowl, mix the cauliflower with the garlic. Pulse until the finely chopped like a fine meal, for around three minutes. Move to a broad blending pot.
- Mix the mozzarella, eggs, thyme, parmesan, egg white, and rosemary in the cauliflower until well blended; add salt and pepper.
- Spread the cauliflower mixture in a 1/2-inch-thick ring upon the baking sheet. Brush the olive oil on the surface. Bake until the sides are crisp and light golden, for 25 to 30 minutes.
- Cool for five min before cutting and able to serve in the sticks.

5. Rainbow Dinner Keto Chicken

Servings: 4 | Total time: 45 min

Calories: 394 kcal | Proteins: 39 g | Carbohydrates: 23 g | Fat: 16 g

Ingredients

- Nonstick spray
- One-pound chicken
- One tablespoon sesame oil
- Two tablespoons soy sauce
- Two tablespoons honey
- Two diced red bell peppers
- Two diced yellow bell peppers
- Three sliced carrots
- Half broccoli
- Two diced red onions
- Two tablespoons of olive oil
- A pinch of Kosher salt and black pepper
- One fourth cup chopped parsley

Steps of preparation

- Begin by Preheating the oven to a temperature of 400 ° F. Spray a baking sheet slightly with a nonstick spray.
- Put the chicken upon this baking sheet. In a bowl, shake with the sesame oil and the soy sauce. Brush the paste uniformly with the chicken.
- Place the red bell peppers, the yellow bell peppers, the vegetables, the broccoli, and the red onion on a baking sheet. Sprinkle the olive oil all over the vegetables and stir gently to coat, now season with some salt and pepper.
- Bake until the vegetables are soft as well as the chicken is thoroughly cooked for 23 to 25 minutes. Pull the mixture from oven and season with parsley.

6. Keto Dinner Chicken Meatballs

Servings: 4 | Total time: 45 min

Calories: 205 kcal | Proteins: 20 g | Carbohydrates: 3 g | Fat: 13 g

Ingredients

- One tablespoon olive oil
- Half chopped red onion
- 2 tablespoon minced garlic
- One-pound ground chicken
- One fourth cup chopped fresh parsley
- One tablespoon mustard paste
- Three fourth teaspoon kosher salt
- Half teaspoon black pepper
- One can coconut milk
- One and ¼ cups fresh parsley chopped
- Four chopped scallions
- One garlic minced
- One lemon zest and juice
- A pinch of Kosher salt and black pepper
- A pinch of Red pepper flakes
- One recipe Cauliflower Rice

Steps of preparation

- Start by Preheating the oven to 375 ° F. Lay a baking sheet with an aluminum foil and coat this with a non - stick cooking spray.
- Heat the olive oil in a medium skillet over medium heat. Include the onion and sauté until soft, for about five minutes. Include the garlic and sauté until fragrant for around 1 minute.

- Move the garlic and the onion to a medium bowl and let it cool moderately. Stir in parsley, chicken, and the mustard, sprinkle in pepper and salt. Shape the mixture into 2 tablespoon spheres and shift to the baking sheet.
- Bake the meatballs unless solid and thoroughly cooked for 17 to 20 mins.
- In a food processor jar, mix parsley, scallions, garlic, coconut milk, lemon zest, and lemon juice and mix thoroughly, sprinkle with salt and black pepper.
- Cover with both the red pepper flakes as well as the remaining parsley. Serve the sauce over cauliflower rice.

7. Keto Dinner Pork Carnitas

Servings: 4 | Total time: 45 min

Calories: 205 kcal | Proteins: 20 g | Carbohydrates: 3 g | Fat: 13 g

Ingredients

- One sliced white onion
- Five minced garlic cloves
- One minced jalapeño
- Three pounds pork shoulder (diced)
- A pinch of salt and black pepper
- One tablespoon cumin
- Two tablespoons fresh oregano
- Two oranges

- One lime
- One-third cup of chicken broth

Steps of preparation

- Put the onion, garlic, the jalapeno, and the pork at the bottom of the slow cooker. Put cinnamon, oregano pepper, and cumin to taste.
- Put the oranges and lime zest all over the pork, and then halve them and drop the juice all over the pork. Spill the broth over the pork as well.
- Place the cover on the slow cooker and hold the heat down. Cook for almost 7 hours or till meat is soft and quick to break with a fork.
- Utilize two forks to crumble the beef. Pork may be presented immediately (we like it in tacos) or frozen in an airtight jar in a refrigerator for up to 5 days or in a freezer for up to 1 month.

8. Keto Butter Scallops Garlic and Steak

Servings: 4 | Total time: 45 min

Calories: 205 kcal | Proteins: 20 g | Carbohydrates: 3 g | Fat: 13 g

Ingredients

- Two beef tenderloin fillets
- A pinch of Kosher salt and black pepper
- Three tablespoons unsalted butter

- Eight to ten large sea scallops
- Three minced garlic cloves
- Six tablespoons cubed unsalted butter
- Two tablespoons parsley leaves chopped
- Two tablespoons fresh chives
- One tablespoon lemon juice
- Two teaspoons lemon zest
- A pinch of Kosher salt and black pepper

Steps of preparation

- Warm a cast iron pan on a medium-high flame for ten minutes.
- Use paper towels, pat all sides of steak dry; spice with some salt and pepper as you want.
- Melt 2 tbsp of butter. Put the steaks in the center of the pan and cook for around 4-6 mins until the thick crust has developed. Use tongs, flip and simmer for another five minutes or until done as desired; set the pan aside, cover it loosely.
- As the steak rests, clean the steak and heat the leftover one tablespoon of butter into it.
- Strip the short side muscle from of the scallops, clean with cold water, and dry completely.
- Season with salt and black pepper. Work in rounds, add the scallops to the pan in a single layer and fry, flip once, till golden brown and transparent in the middle,

approximately three minutes per side. Put aside and leave it warm.

- o Reducing overall heat to low for garlic butter sauce; add the garlic and simmer, stir constantly, until fragrant, for around 1 minute. Stir in butter, chives, lemon juice, parsley, and lemon zest, now season with salt and pepper.
- o In the end, serve steaks and scallops directly with the garlic butter sauce.

9. Ketogenic Cauliflower Crispy Wrapped Prosciutto Bites

Servings: 8-10 | Total time: 45 min

Calories: 215 kcal | Proteins: 14 g | Carbohydrates: 5 g | Fat: 15 g

Ingredients

- o One small head cauliflower
- o Half cup tomato paste
- o Two tablespoons white wine
- o Half teaspoon black pepper
- o Half cup grated Parmesan cheese
- o Twenty slices prosciutto
- o Six tablespoons olive oil

Steps of preparation

- o Cut the bottom of the cauliflower and some green leaves. Split the cauliflower in half and slice the half into one-inch-thick strips. Split the slices into two or three bits, based on the size of the slice.

- o Put to a boil a big pot of salted water. Blanch the cauliflower in water until it is almost soft, for 3 to 5 minutes. Remove the cauliflower and pat dry with the help of paper towels.
- o In a small cup, combine the tomato paste with black pepper and white wine. Layer 1 tsp along each side of the cauliflower, then top with 1 tsp of Parmesan. Gently seal a prosciutto slice over each piece of the cauliflower, gripping gently at the end to secure
- o Work in batches, cook two teaspoons of olive oil in a wide pan over medium heat. Bring the cauliflower then cook till the prosciutto is crispy and golden, three to four minutes per side. Then repeat with some extra oil and cauliflower until all the bits are fried. Let it settle slowly, then serve.

10. Ketogenic Fried Chicken Recipe

Servings: 12 | Total time: 12 min

Calories: 308 kcal | Proteins: 40.4 g | Carbohydrates: 0.7 g | Fat: 14 g

Ingredients

- o Four ounces of pork rinds
- o One and a half teaspoon thyme dried
- o One teaspoon sea salt dried
- o One teaspoon black pepper dried

- o One teaspoon oregano dried
- o Half teaspoon garlic powder dried
- o One teaspoon paprika dried
- o Twelve chicken legs and thighs
- o One egg
- o Two ounces mayonnaise
- o Three tablespoons of mustard

Steps of preparation

- o Start by preheating the oven at a temperature of 400 degrees Fahrenheit.
- o Grind pork rinds in a powder form, leaving them in a few bigger pieces.
- o Mix pork rinds with thyme, pepper, oregano, salt, garlic, and smoked paprika. Spread on a large plate into a thin sheet.
- o In a big container, mix egg, mayonnaise, and Dijon mustard. Dip every piece of chicken in the egg-mayonnaise mixture, and then wrap in the pork rind blend until it is thinly coated.
- o Put the chicken on a wire rack on a baking sheet and then bake for almost 40 minutes.

11. Greek Yogurt Chicken Peppers salad

Servings: 6 | Total time: 30 min

Calories: 116 kcal | Proteins: 7 g | Carbohydrates: 16 g | Fat: 3 g

Ingredients

- o Two-third cup of Greek yogurt
- o Two tablespoons mustard paste
- o Two tablespoons vinegar
- o A pinch of Kosher salt and black pepper
- o One-third cup of chopped fresh parsley
- o Half kg of cubed roseate chicken
- o Two sliced stalks celery
- o One bunch of sliced scallions
- o One pint of cherry tomatoes
- o Half diced cucumber
- o Three bell peppers

Steps of preparation

- o In a bowl, combine Greek yogurt, and rice vinegar, and mustard; add salt and pepper. Put some parsley.
- o Include chicken, celery and three - fourths of the scallions, and cucumbers and tomatoes. Stir well and mix.
- o Distribute the chicken salad between the bell peppers.
- o Garnish the remainder scallions, some tomatoes, and cucumbers.

12. Easy chicken low carb stir fry recipe

Serving: 2| Total Time: 12 mins

Calories: 219 | Fat:10g |Net Carbs:5.5g |Protein:19g

Ingredients

- Sesame oil 1 tbsp
- Boneless & skinless chicken thighs 2
- Minced fresh ginger 1 Tbsp
- Gluten-free soy sauce 1/4 cup
- Water 1/2 cup
- Onion powder 1 tsp
- Garlic powder 1/2 tsp
- Red pepper flakes 1 tsp
- Granulated sugar1 Tbsp
- Xanthan gum 1/2 tsp
- Bagged broccolis mix 2 heaping cups
- Chopped scallions 1/2 cup

Steps of Preparation

- Cut the chicken thighs into thin pieces/strips. Mix the chicken & chopped ginger in the edible oil in a big sauté pan for 2 to 3 mins.
- Apply the water, soy sauce, powder of onion, powder of garlic, red pepper flakes, sugar sub & xanthan gum. Remove well and simmer for five mins.
- Apply the slaw & scallions then coat — simmer for two min.

13. Keto Asiago Chicken with Bacon Cream Sauce

Serving: 4 | Total Time: 40 mins

Calories 581 kcal | Fat:38g | Net Carbs:8g | Protein:49g

Ingredients

- Chicken breasts 1.5 lb.
- Vegetable oil 1 1/2 tbsp
- Salt & pepper
- Minced garlic cloves 4
- Chicken stock 1 cup
- Cooked & chopped bacon 8 slices
- Sliced lemon 1/2
- Half & half 1 cup
- Shredded asiago cheese 1/2 cup
- Fresh chopped parsley 2 tbsp

Steps of Preparation

- Season the chicken nicely with salt & pepper on each side. Heat the vegetable fats in the big pan. Roast the chicken breasts over med-high heat- around two mins on per side to brown a bit. Do not cook the chicken thru-you will continue to cook it afterward. Take away the chicken from your Pan.
- Add chopped garlic to the same pan. Cook on med heat for around thirty sec, scraping the bottom of the skillet. Deglaze the skillet with a little chicken stock. Apply the leftover stock (total 1 cup).
- Apply half the bacon to the chicken broth.
- Return the chicken to the saucepan, on top of the bacon, as well as in the broth of the chicken. Prepare 5 slim lemon slices across the breasts of the chicken and cook, boiling at low heat, covered for around

twenty mins, till the chicken is fully cooked & no longer pink in the middle.

o Take away the chicken from the pan after it is fully cooked. Remove the slices of lemon from the pan. It is much important to remove them. Do not abandon them in for the sauce, or else it'll be too sour. Put one half-and-a-half cup to the pan. Bring to the boil & stir well, scrap from the bottom. Apply 1/2 cup of Asiago shredded cheese & mix to melt totally, just around thirty sec.

o Spoon a little sauce on the chicken breasts to serve & toss with the leftover minced bacon & minced parsley.

14. Ketogenic Grilled Chicken Souvlaki with Yogurt Sauce

Serving 4 | Total Time: 2hour 10 mins |

Calories: 192 | Fat:7g | Net Carbs:2.5g | Protein:27g

Ingredients

o Chicken breast (cut in strips) 1 lb.

o Olive oil 3 tbsp

o Lemon juice 3 tbsp

o Red wine vinegar 1 tbsp

o Fresh chopped oregano 1 tbsp

o Minced garlic 4 cloves

o Kosher salt 2 tsp

o Ground black pepper 1/4 tsp

o Dried thyme 1/2 tsp

For the yogurt sauce

o Greek yogurt 3/4 cup

o Lemon juice 1 tsp

o Minced Garlic 1 tsp

o Fresh chopped oregano 1 tsp

o Kosher salt 1/2 tsp

o Granulated sugar 1/2 tsp

Steps of Preparation

o In a small non-reactive bowl, mix the oil of olive, juice of lemon, red vinegar, garlic, oregano, pepper, salt, & dried thyme.

o Fill the marinade with the chicken strips and combine well to cover.

o Cover in the freezer & marinate for two hours or longer.

o Take away the chicken from marinade & thread (when using) on skewers.

o Heat the grill & grill the chicken for around two mins each side, or when it is cooked thru.

For the yogurt sauce:

o Mix all the ingredients of the yogurt sauce & mix well. Season it with your preference.

o Serve the hot grilled chicken with them.

15. Low Carb Chicken Jalapeño Poppers

Serving 15 | Total Time: 30 mins

Calories: 111 | Fat:9g |Net Carbs:1g |Protein:1g

Ingredients

- Jalapenos large 15
- Sharp shredded cheddar cheese 1 cup
- Softened cream cheese 8 oz
- Shredded & chopped cooked chicken 2 cups
- Salsa Verde 1/3 cup
- Garlic powder 1/2 tsp
- Kosher salt 1/2 tsp
- Cajun seasoning 1 tsp
- Pulverized pork rinds 1 cup
- Cajun seasoning 1/2 tsp

Steps of Preparation

- Slice each pepper one/three off the top & scoop out in there.
- Put the peppers on a tray & microwave to soften for two mins.
- In a med bowl, mix cream cheese, cheddar cheese, chicken/turkey, salsa Verde, powder of garlic, salt & Cajun seasoning, then mix till it's blended & creamy.
- Spoon the blend within the jalapeños.
- Mix the pork rind powder & Cajun seasoning in a tiny bowl.
- Nicely roll the cream cheese part of the filled jalapeños into the rinds of Cajun pork till covered.
- Put on the baking sheet.
- Cook for twenty mins at 400, or till its color changes to golden brown & bubble.
- Cool before serving, for a minimum of five mins.

16. Lemon butter chicken

Total Time: 50 mins | Serving: 8

Ingredients

- Chicken thighs 8 bone
- Smoked paprika 1 tbsp
- Ground black pepper & kosher salt
- Divided unsalted butter 3 tbsp
- Minced garlic 3 cloves
- Chicken broth 1 cup
- Heavy cream 1/2 cup
- Freshly grated parmesan 1/4 cup
- Lemon juice 1
- Dried thyme 1 tsp
- Chopped baby spinach 2 cups

Steps of Preparation

- Oven Preheated to 205 degrees C.
- Top chicken thighs with salt, paprika & pepper.

- Melt two tbsp of butter on med-high heat in a big oven-proof pan. Put chicken, skin side down, & sear on each side till they become golden brown, approximately 2 to 3 mins each side; sink excess fat & set it aside.
- Melt the remaining tbsp of butter in the pan. Apply the garlic & cook till fragrant, constantly whisking, approximately 1 to 2 mins, mix in chicken broth, whipping cream, parmesan, juice of lemon, and thyme.
- Bring to a boil; lower the heat, mix in the spinach & boil till the spinach had also wilted & the sauce had already thickened slightly around 3 to 5 mins.
- Put in the oven & roast for around 25 to 30 min till fully cooked, trying to reach a core temp of 75 degrees C.
- Serve asap.

17. Keto Chicken Low Carb Stir Fry.

Servings: 4 | Total time: 22 min

Calories: 116 kcal | Proteins: 28 g | Carbohydrates: 9 g | Fat: 7 g

Ingredients

- One fourth Olive oil
- One-pound Chicken breast
- Half teaspoon sea salt
- One by four teaspoon Black pepper
- Four Garlic minced
- Six ounces of Broccoli
- One Red bell pepper
- One fourth cup Chicken bone broth
- One-pound Cauliflower rice
- One fourth Coconut aminos
- One teaspoon Toasted sesame oil
- One fourth cup green onions

Steps of preparation

- Heat 2 tablespoons of olive oil in a large pan over medium heat. Include the strips of chicken and add salt and pepper. Now cook for 4-5 minutes, turning once, until chicken is crispy and just cooked thru.
- Remove the chicken from the pan, set it aside, then cover to keep it warm.
- Apply the remaining two tbsp (30 ml) of olive oil in a pan. Include the crushed garlic and then sauté for around a minute until aromatic.
- Include the broccoli and the bell pepper. Cook for 3-4 minutes before the broccoli begins to turn bright green, and the peppers tend to soften.
- Add the broth of bone. To deglaze, scrape the base of the pan. Reduce to medium temperature. Cover the pan and

simmer for 3-5 minutes, until the broccoli is crisp.

○ Transfer coconut aminos to pan, scrape the bottom of the pan and deglaze again. Put the chicken back in the pan. Transfer the rice to the cauliflower. Heat up to medium-high again. Now Stir for 3-4 minutes, before the cauliflower is tender but not mushy, most liquid evaporates, and the chicken is fully cooked through.

○ Remove from the heat. Cover in toasted sesame oil. Add salt and black pepper if necessary. Cover with green onion, as needed

18. Keto Tomato chicken zoodles

Servings: 4 | Total time: 20 min

Calories: 411 kcal | Proteins: 45 g | Carbohydrates: 11 g | Fat: 18.8 g

Ingredients

○ Coconut butter ½ tsp
○ Diced onion 1 medium
○ Chicken fillets 450- 500 g
○ Garlic clove, 1 minced
○ Zucchinis two medium
○ Crushed tomatoes 400 g
○ Chop half 7-10 cherry tomatoes
○ Cashews 100 g
○ Salt

○ Dry oregano & basil
○ Black pepper

Steps of preparation

○ Heat a wide pan over medium heat. Add the coconut butter and the sliced onion. Cook for about 30 seconds to about 1 minute. Be alert, so you don't roast the onions.

○ Slice the chicken into 2 cm chunks.

○ Apply chicken and garlic to the pan. Season with the basil, the oregano salt and black pepper. Cook the chicken for about 5-6 minutes each side.

○ Spiralize the zucchini when the chicken is frying. Cut them short when they're wanted. Use the vegetable peeler to create the ribbons out from the zucchini.

○ Add the crushed tomatoes and simmer for about 3-5 minutes.

○ Cook the cashews in another pan until golden brown. Taste and adjust with paprika, some turmeric and salt.

○ Now add the spiralled zoodles, some cherry tomatoes and sprinkle with extra salt as appropriate. Cook for the next 1 minute and then switch off the heat.

○ Now serve chicken zoodles with crispy cashews and the fresh basil.

19. Tuscan garlic chicken

Servings: 6 | Total time: 25 min

Calories: 225 kcal | Proteins: 30 g | Carbohydrates: 7 g | Fat: 25 g

Ingredients

- Boneless chicken breasts 1½ pounds
- Olive oil 2 Tablespoons
- Heavy cream 1 cup
- Chicken broth 1/2 cup
- Garlic powder 1 teaspoon
- Italian seasoning 1 teaspoon
- Parmesan cheese 1/2 cup
- Chopped spinach 1 cup
- Dried tomatoes 1/2 cup

Steps of Preparation

- Put olive oil in a wide skillet and cook chicken on medium heat for about 3-5 minutes on every side or until it gets brown on each side and then cook until the middle is no longer pink. Remove the chicken and put it aside on a tray.
- Include some of the chicken broth, the garlic powder, the heavy cream, the Italian seasoning and also some parmesan cheese. Simmer over on a medium-high flame until it thickens. Include the spinach and the tomatoes and then cook before the spinach becomes soggy. Transfer the chicken onto the plate.
- Serve over pasta.

20. Turkey and peppers

Servings: 4 | Total time: 20 min

Calories: 230 kcal | Proteins: 30 g | Carbohydrates: 11 g | Fat: 8 g

Ingredients

- Salt 1 teaspoon
- Turkey tenderloin 1 pound
- Olive oil 2 tablespoons
- Sliced onion ½ large
- Red bell pepper 1
- Yellow bell pepper 1
- Italian seasoning ½ teaspoon
- Black pepper ¼ teaspoon
- Vinegar 2 teaspoons
- Crushed tomatoes 14-ounce
- Parsley and basil for garnishing

Steps of preparation

- Sprinkle outa ½ teaspoon of salt over the turkey. Heat 1 tablespoon of the oil in a wide non-stick pan over medium heat. Include almost half of the turkey and then cook until golden brown on the rim, for 1 to 3 minutes. Flip and continue to cook for 2 minutes. Now remove the turkey from the slotted spatula to the tray, cover with foil to keep it warm. Apply the remaining 1 tablespoon of oil to the pan, reduce the heat to low and then repeat with the remaining turkey for 1 to 3 minutes per side.

o Transfer the onion, the bell peppers and the remainder 1/2 teaspoon of the salt to the pan, cover and simmer, then remove the lid and stir often, until the onion and the peppers are softened and golden brown in the spots for almost 5 to 7 minutes.

o Replace the cover, raise the heat to almost medium-high, then sprinkle with Italian seasoning and pepper and roast with stirring constantly before the herbs are fragrant for around 30 seconds. Now add vinegar and then cook until almost fully evaporated, for around 20 seconds. Put tomatoes and bring to a simmer, stirring regularly.

o Transfer the turkey to the pan with any leftover juices and bring to simmer. Now reduce the heat to medium-low and then cook until the turkey is hot all through the sauce for almost 1 to 2 minutes. Serve topped with parsley and basil if it's used.

21. Ketogenic Ginger butter chicken

Servings: 4 | Total time: 20 min

Calories: 293 kcal | Proteins: 29 g | Carbohydrates: 9 g | Fat: 17 g

Ingredients

o Cubed chicken breast 1.5 pounds
o Garam masala 2 tablespoons
o Fresh ginger grated 3 teaspoons
o Minced garlic 3 teaspoons
o Greek yogurt 4 ounces
o Coconut oil 1 tablespoon
o Ghee 2 tablespoons
o Onion sliced 1
o Fresh ginger grated 2 teaspoons
o Minced garlic 2 teaspoons
o Can crushed tomatoes 14.5 oz
o Ground coriander 1 tablespoon
o Garam masala 1/2 tablespoon
o Cumin 2 teaspoons
o Chili powder 1 teaspoon
o Heavy cream 1/2 cup
o Salt
o Cilantro

Instruction

o Slice chicken into 2 inches pieces and put in a wide bowl with 2 teaspoons of garam masala, one teaspoon of fried ginger and one teaspoon of minced garlic. Attach the yogurt, whisk to mix. Transfer to the refrigerator and cool for at least 30 minutes.

o Place the onion, ginger, garlic, and spices and crushed tomatoes in a blender and blend until soft. Set it aside

- Heat 1 tablespoon oil in a wide pan over medium heat. Put chicken and marinade in the pan, fry three to four minutes per side. After browning, add in the sauce and simmer for 5 to 6 minutes.
- Mix in the heavy cream and ghee and proceed to cook for another minute. Taste the salt and apply the extra if necessary. Cover with cilantro and, if needed, serve with some cauliflower rice.

22. Keto BLT Lettuce Wraps

Total Time: 25 minutes | Servings: 4

Calories: Kcal 368 | Fat: 30.8g | Net Carbs: 15.8g | Protein: 11.6g

Ingredients

- From 1 med head butter lettuce 8 leaves, like Bibb or Boston
- Bacon 6 slices
- Mayonnaise 2 tbsp
- Fine chopped chives 1 tbsp
- Squeezed freshly lemon juice 1 tbsp
- Black pepper ground freshly 1/8 tsp
- Grape tomatoes half or pint cherry 1
- Diced avocado 1 med

Steps of Preparation

- Set up a rack in the bottom third of the oven and to 400 ° F heat it. Lined a baking sheet with an aluminum foil or parchment paper.
- Place the bacon in one layer onto the baking sheet. Bake 15 to 20 mins until crispy and rich golden-brown. From the oven, Remove and allow cool. Alternatively, in a shallow pot, mix the mayonnaise, lemon juice, chives, and pepper; set aside.
- Move the bacon to a cutting board until it's cold and chop it roughly. Load a single leaf of lettuce with tomatoes, avocado, and bacon. Drizzle with the dressing, then serve.

23. Chipotle Avocado Mayonnaise

Total Time: 5 minutes | Serving 1

Calories Kcal 188 | Fat: 18.9g | Net Carbs: 5.8g | Protein: 1.4g

Ingredients

- Medium avocados 2 ripe
- Chipotle chile canned finely chopped in adobo sauce 1 tsp
- Dijon mustard 1 tsp
- Lemon juice freshly squeezed 1 tsp
- Kosher salt 1/2 tsp
- Olive oil 1/4 cup

Steps of Preparation

- In a mini food processor or blender, place the chipotle chili, avocados, in adobo sauce, lemon juice, Dijon mustard, and kosher salt. Process till smooth, for 30 - 1 minute. Scrape the bowl or pitcher side. Switch on the machine and drizzle gradually into the oil. Blend, about 1 minute, till smooth & emulsified.

24. Keto Egg Dinner Muffins

Total Time:15 minutes | Serving 12 muffins

Calories: Kcal 227 | Fat: 7.3g | Net Carbs: 5.3g| Protein: 11.7g

Ingredients

- Olive oil or Cooking spray
- Sweet potato shredded 1 1/2 cups
- Cheddar cheese shredded sharp 1 cup
- Strips bacon sugar-free, crumbled 6 cooked
- Large eggs 10
- Kosher salt 1 teaspoon
- Black pepper freshly ground 1/4 tsp

Steps of Preparation

- Arrange a middle-rack in -oven and to 400 ° F heat. Coat a regular 12 well muffin tray generously with olive oil or cooking spray. Divide the sliced sweet potato, bacon, and cheese equally throughout the wells of muffins.

- In a big cup, put the eggs, half-&-a-half, pepper, and salt and whisk till the eggs are thoroughly integrated. Pour in the wells of the muffins, filling 1/2 to 3/4 complete each.
- Bake for 12 - 14 minutes, till the muffins, are set and brown slightly around edges. On a wire rack, place the pan and allow it to cool for 2 - 3 mins. Run the butter knife to the release of the muffins around cups each of them before extracting them. Serve cold or warm, before cooling or freezing, absolutely on a wire rack.

25. Prosciutto-Wrapped Avocado with Arugula and Goat Cheese

Total Time: 15 minutes | Servings 4

Calories: Kcal 295 | Fat: 23.1 | Net Carbs: 9.6g| Protein: 15.4g

Ingredients

- Goat cheese fresh 4 ounces
- Lemon juice freshly squeezed 2 tbsp
- Black pepper freshly ground 1/2 tsp
- Kosher salt 1/4 tsp
- Prosciutto 8 thin slices
- Arugula 1 1/2 cups
- Thinly sliced avocados ripe medium 2

Steps of Preparation

o In a shallow pot, mix the goat cheese, lemon juice, salt, and pepper until smooth. Place pieces of the prosciutto. Layer single slice of prosciutto with 2 - 3 tsp of goat cheese mixture. Split the arugula into the prosciutto, placing the greens on one end of each piece. Cover each pile of greens similarly with 2–3 slices of avocado. Operating with one prosciutto slice at a time, then wrapping up into a compact package beginning with the avocado from the end.

26. Garlic Butter Steak Bites

Total Time: 20 minutes | Serving: 2-4

Calories: Kcal 748 | Fat: 61.9g | Net Carbs: 1.4g | Protein: 44.4g

Ingredients

o Garlic 4 cloves
o Black pepper freshly ground 1/2 teaspoon
o Parsley leaves chopped fresh 1/4 cup
o Thick-cut strip steaks New York 2 pounds
o Kosher salt 1/2 teaspoon
o Unsalted butter 8 tablespoons

Steps of Preparation

o Mince 4 cloves of garlic. Place in a cup and apply 1/2 tsp of black pepper freshly ground. Cut until 1/4 cup of fresh parsley leaves is available, then

move to a small pot. Cut 2 pounds of strip steak New York into 1-inch pieces, then apply 1/2 tsp of kosher salt to season.

o Melt 8 tbsp (1 stick) of unsalted butter over medium-high heat in a large skillet. Attach the steak cubes then sear till browned, tossing them halfway through, taking 6 - 8 mins. Add the pepper and garlic, and simmer for another 1 minute. Take off the heat and with the parsley garnish.

27. Pesto Chicken with Burst Cherry Tomatoes

Total Time: 25-30 minutes | Serving 4

Calories: Kcal 445 | Fat: 16.2g | Net Carbs: 8.2g | Protein: 63.6g

Ingredients

o Grape tomatoes or pints cherry 2
o Olive oil 1 tbsp
o Kosher salt 1/2 tsp
o Black pepper freshly ground 1/4 tsp
o Chicken breasts boneless, skinless 4
o Basil pesto 1/4 cup

Steps of Preparation

o Place a rack in the center of the oven and to 400 ° F heat the oven.
o Put the tomatoes on a baking sheet, which is rimmed. Remove the grease, season

with pepper and salt, and mix. Spread out over a single sheet.

o Pat, the chicken, completely dries it with paper towels. Season with pepper and salt. Put the chicken on the baking sheet in the middle. Spread the pesto on each chicken breast (about 1 tbsp each), spread on a thin layer, so each breast is covered evenly and fully.

o Roast until caramelized the tomatoes have, and others have burst and cooked the chicken and registers 165 ° F, 25 - 30 mins, on a thermometer. Serve the drizzled chicken and tomatoes with pan juices.

28. Scrambled eggs with basil and butter

Total Time: 10 mins | Serving 1

Calories: Kcal 641 | Fat:59g | Net Carbs:3g | Protein:26g

Ingredients

o Butter 2 tbsp
o Eggs 2
o Heavy whipping cream 2 tbsp
o Ground black pepper & salt
o Shredded cheese 2 oz
o Fresh basil 2 tbsp

Steps of Preparation

o Melt butter over low heat in a saucepan.

o In a small cup, put cracked eggs, shredded cheese, cream, and seasoning. Offer it a quick whisk and apply it to the saucepan.

o Push from the side to the middle with a spatula before the eggs are scrambled. If you want fluffy and soft, mix on lower heat to desired consistency.

29. Keto seafood special omelet

Total Time: 20 mins | Serving 2

Calories: Kcal 872 | Fat:83g | Net Carbs:4g | Protein:27g

Ingredients

o Olive oil 2 tbsp
o Cooked shrimp 5 oz
o Red chili pepper 1
o ½ tsp fennel seeds or ground cumin
o Mayonnaise ½ cup
o Fresh chives 1 tbsp
o Eggs 6
o Olive oil 2 tbsp
o Salt & pepper

Steps of Preparation

o Preheat the broiler.

o In olive oil, broil the seafood or shrimp mixture with the chopped garlic, chili, cumin, fennel seeds, salt & pepper.

o To cooled seafood mixture, apply mayo and chives.

- o Whisk the eggs together, season with salt & pepper, and cook in a non-stick saucepan with butter or oil.
- o When the omelet is nearly full, apply the seafood mixture. Fold. Reduce the heat and enable it to set fully. Serve.

30. Keto Fried eggs

Total Time: 10 mins | Serving 4

Per serving: Kcal 226, Fat:20g, Net Carbs:1g Protein:11g

Ingredients

- o Butter 4 tbsp
- o Eggs 8
- o Salt & pepper

Steps of Preparation

- o Heat coconut oil or butter over medium heat in a frying pan.
- o Break the eggs directly into the saucepan. For sunny side up eggs, allow the eggs to be fried on one side. Cover the saucepan with a lid to ensure that they are fried on top. For eggs that are easily cooked, turn over the eggs after a few mins and then cook for another.
- o Season with salt & pepper.

31. Keto egg butter with smoked salmon and avocado

Total Time: 20 mins | Serving 2

Calories: 1148, Fat:112g, Net Carbs:5g Protein:26g

Ingredients

- o Eggs 4
- o Sea salt ½ tsp
- o Ground black pepper ¼ tsp
- o Butter 5 oz
- o Avocados 2
- o Olive oil 2 tbsp
- o Chopped fresh parsley 1 tbsp
- o Smoked salmon 4 oz

Steps of Preparation

- o Carefully put the eggs in a pot. Cover with colder water and place without the lid on the stove. Get the water to boil.
- o Reduce heat and allow to simmer for 7-8 mins, from the warmed water. Remove the eggs and put them in an ice-cold bowl to cool.
- o Peel and chop the eggs completely. Combine the eggs with the butter with the fork. Season with the pepper, salt, and other spices of your choosing
- o Serve.

32. Ketogenic scallions egg muffins

Total Time: 25 mins | Serving 6

Calories: Kcal 336, Fat:26g, Net Carbs:2g Protein:23g

Ingredients

- Finely chopped scallions 2
- Chopped air-dried chorizo 5 oz.
- Eggs 12
- Salt & pepper
- Shredded cheese 6 oz

Steps of Preparation

- Preheat an oven to 175 ° C (350 ° F).
- Line a non-stick muffin tray with insertable baking cups/grease, a buttered silicone muffin tin.
- Apply the chorizo and scallions to the tin base.
- Mix the eggs with the pesto, pepper, and salt then incorporate the cheese and mix.
- Pour the batter over the scallions and the chorizo.
- Bake the muffin tin for 15–20 mins, depending on the scale.

33. Keto fried eggs with kale and pork

Total Time:20 mins | Serving 2

Calories: Kcal 1033, Fat:99g, Net Carbs:8g Protein:26g

Ingredients

- Kale ½ lb.
- Butter 3 oz
- Smoked pork belly 6 oz

- Frozen cranberries 1 oz
- Pecans 1 oz.
- Eggs 4
- Salt & pepper

Steps of Preparation

- Chop and Trim the kale into wide squares. Melt 2/3rd of the butter in the frying pan and cook the kale rapidly over high heat until the sides are slightly browned.
- From the frying pan, Remove the kale and put aside. Cook the bacon or pork belly in the frying pan until it is crisp.
- Reduce heat. The sautéed kale is Returned to the saucepan and add the nuts and cranberries. Remove until soft
- Turn the flame on the rest of the butter and fry the eggs. Add Salt and pepper. Put two fried eggs for each part of the greens and serve.

34. Keto Croque Monsieur

Total Time: 20 mins | Serving 2

Calories: Kcal 1083, Fat:92g, Net Carbs:8g Protein:54g

Ingredients

- Cottage cheese 8 oz
- Eggs 4
- Husk powder ground psyllium 1 tbsp
- Butter 4 tbsp
- deli ham 5⅓ oz

- Cheddar cheese 5 1/3 oz
- Lettuce 3½ oz.
- Olive oil 4 tbsp
- Red wine vinegar ½ tbsp
- Salt & pepper

Steps of Preparation

- In a bowl, whisk the eggs. Blend in cottage cheese. Apply a psyllium husk powder ground when stirring in order incorporate it without lumps smoothly. Rest the mixture for five minutes before the batter has formed.
- Put the frying pan over med heat. Apply a large quantity of butter and cook the batter like tiny pancakes on either side for a few minutes, until they are brown.
- Create a sandwich between the two warm pancakes with cheese and sliced ham. Add finely diced onion on top.
- Wash and cut the lettuce. In a clear vinaigrette, add the oil, vinegar, salt, and pepper.

35. Veggie keto scramble

Total Time: 20 mins | Serving 1

Calories: Kcal 415, Fat:31g, Net Carbs:4g Protein:28g

Ingredients

- Butter 1 tbsp
- Sliced mushrooms 1 oz.

- Eggs 3
- Diced red bell peppers 1 oz
- Ground black pepper & salt
- Shredded parmesan cheese 1 oz
- Chopped scallion ½

Steps of Preparation

- Heat the butter over medium heat in a wide frying pan. Add the sliced mushrooms, diced red peppers, salt, and fry until tender.
- Put the eggs directly into the saucepan and quickly mix so that it is properly incorporated.
- Transfer the spatula to create big, soft curds over the bottom and side of the skillet. Cook until no clear liquid egg remains.
- Put the scramble with scallions and shredded parmesan on top.

36. Keto dinner chaffles

Time: 25 mins | Serving 4

Calories: Kcal 599, Fat:50g, Net Carbs:4g Protein:32g

Ingredients

- Eggs 4
- Shredded cheddar cheese 8 oz
- Chopped fresh chives 2 tbsp
- Salt & pepper

Toppings

- Eggs 4
- Sliced bacon 8
- Sliced cherry tomatoes 8
- Baby spinach 2 oz

Steps of Preparation

- Heat the waffle maker.
- Place the bacon slices in a big, unheated frying pan and raise the temperature to med heat. Cook the bacon for around 8-12 mins, regularly rotating, until it is crispy to taste.
- Set aside to cool as you cook the chaffles on a paper towel.
- Put all ingredients of your waffle in a mixing bowl & beat to blend.
- Grind the waffle iron lightly and spoon the mixture equally over the bottom surface, spreading it out to achieve an even outcome.
- Shut the waffle iron then cook according to the waffle maker for approx. 6 mins.
- Break the eggs in the bacon grease in the frying pan as the chaffles are heating, then cook softly until finished.
- Serve with scrambled egg and baby spinach, bacon strips, and cherry tomatoes on each chaffles side.

Chapter 5: Keto snacks recipes for women above 50

1. Keto Tortilla Chips

Servings: 10 chips | Total time: 40 min

Calories: 198 kcal | Proteins: 11 g | Carbohydrates: 4 g | Fat: 16 g

Ingredients

o shredded mozzarella 2 cups
o almond flour 1 cups
o kosher salt 1 teaspoon
o garlic powder 1 teaspoon
o chili powder half teaspoon
o Black pepper

Steps of preparation

o Preheat the oven to 350 ° F. Place two big baking sheets of parchment paper.

o Melt mozzarella in a microwave safe jar, around 1 minute and 30 seconds. Include almond flour, cinnamon, garlic powder, chili powder and several cracks of black pepper. Use your hands to knead the dough a few times until the ball is smooth.

o Put the dough between the two sheets of the parchment paper and then roll it into a rectangle 1/8 "wide. Break the dough into triangles by using a knife.

o Scatter the chips on the lined baking sheets and cook until the sides are crispy and begin to be crisp, for 12 to 14 minutes.

2. Ketogenic Avocado Chips

Servings: 6 chips | Total time: 30 min

Calories: 171 kcal | Proteins: 7 g | Carbohydrates: 6 g | Fat: 16 g

Ingredients

o Ripe avocado 1 large
o Freshly grated parmesan 3/4 cup.
o Lemon juice 1 teaspoon
o Garlic powder half teaspoon
o Italian seasoning half teaspoon
o A pinch of kosher salt
o Black pepper

Steps of preparation

o Start by Preheating the oven to 325 ° f and then line two baking sheets with a parchment paper. In a medium dish, mash the avocado with a fork until it is smooth. Stir in Parmesan, some lemon juice, some garlic powder and also Italian seasonings. Season with salt and pepper.

o Put the heaping teaspoon-sized mixture scoops on the baking sheet, leaving around 3 "apart across each scoop. Deflate each scoop to 3 "wide with the wooden spoon or a cup. Now bake it until it is crispy and golden, for about 30 minutes, then let it cool to room temperature. Serve at room temperature.

o

3. Ketogenic Nacho Cheese Crisps

Servings: 9 chips | Total time: 1 hr. min

Calories:99 kcal | Proteins: 6 g | Carbohydrates:1.3 g | Fat: 7 g

Ingredients

o Sliced cheddar 8-oz.
o Taco seasoning 2 tsp.

Steps of preparation

o Start by preheating the oven to 250° and then line a baking sheet with a parchment paper. Now cut slices of cheese into about 9 squares and then place them in a medium bowl. Now add the taco seasoning.

o Put cheese slices on the prepared baking sheet. Now bake them until crisp and golden brown, for about 40 minutes. Let them cool for 10 minutes and then remove from the parchment paper.

4. Ketogenic coconut vanilla Ice Cream

Servings: 3 | Total time: 10 min

Calories: 347 kcal | Proteins: 2 g | Carbohydrates: 3 g | Fat: 36 g

Ingredients

o Coconut milk 15-oz.
o Heavy cream 2 cup
o Swerve sweetener 1/4 cup
o Vanilla extract 1 tsp.
o A Pinch of kosher salt

Steps of preparation

o Start by chilling the coconut milk in the refrigerator for about 3 hours, preferably overnight.

o place the coconut cream in a big tub, leave the liquid in a can, using a hand blender to beat the coconut cream till it is very smooth. Set it back.

o Beat heavy cream in a separate wide bowl using a hand blender (or a stand mixer in a bowl) until soft peaks are created. Beat the sweetener and the vanilla.

o Fold the mixed coconut into the whipped cream, then move the mixture to the loaf tray.

o Freeze to a solid condition, around 5 hours.

5. Jalapeno popping Egg Cups

Servings: 12 cups | Total time: 45 min

Calories: 157 kcal | Proteins: 9.7 g | Carbohydrates: 1.3 g | Fat: 9.7 g

Ingredients

- ○ bacon 12 slices
- ○ large eggs 10
- ○ sour cream 1/4 c.
- ○ shredded cheddar half c.
- ○ shredded mozzarella half c.
- ○ sliced 2 jalapeños
- ○ a pinch of kosher salt
- ○ black pepper
- ○ cooking spray

Steps of preparation

- ○ Start by preheating the oven to 375° F. Cook bacon till it becomes slightly browned in a large pan over a medium flame, to drain, set it aside on a plate lined with paper towel.
- ○ In a separate bowl, mix the eggs together with cheeses, minced jalapeño, sour cream, and garlic powder. Now season with salt and pepper.
- ○ Grease a muffin tin through nonstick cooking spray. Put a slice of bacon and line each well, put egg mixture into every muffin cup. Garnish each muffin with a jalapeño slice.
- ○ Now bake for almost 20 minutes, or till the eggs are no longer looking wet. Now Cool them slightly.
- ○ Remove from the muffin tin and serve.

6. Ketogenic Bacon Guac Bombs

Servings: 1 | Total time: 45 min

Calories: 156 kcal | Proteins: 3.4 g | Carbohydrates: 1.4 g | Fat:15.2 g

Ingredients

- ○ cooked 12 slices bacon
- ○ mashed 2 avocados
- ○ cream cheese 6 oz.
- ○ 1 lime Juice
- ○ minced garlic 1 clove
- ○ minced 1/4 red onion
- ○ jalapeno chopped 1 small
- ○ cumin half tsp.
- ○ Chili powder half tsp.
- ○ A pinch of Kosher salt
- ○ black pepper

Steps of preparation

- ○ In a large bowl, put all the ingredients of the guacamole. Stir until it is mostly smooth and then season with the salt and pepper. Put gently in the refrigerator for almost 30 minutes.
- ○ Put the crumbling bacon on a wide tray. Scoop the guacamole mixture with a little cookie scoop and put in the bacon. Roll to coat the bacon. Repeat before both guacamole and bacon are used. Store in the freezer.

7. Ketogenic TPW White Choc Truffles

Servings: 1 | Total time: 1 hour 15 min

Calories: 102 Kcal, |Fat: 7g |Protein: 7g |
Carbohydrates: 3g

Ingredients

o   Pea Protein 60g

o   Chocolate Fudge 80g

o   Syrup Honey flavor 10g

o   dark chocolate 100g

o   chopped salted peanuts 70g

Steps of preparation

o   Mix the pea protein 80, the honey and the stuffed nuts in a wide bowl until mixed. If the mixture is too dry, apply some peanut butter. Apply more protein powder if the combination is too sticky.

o   When your mixture is the consistency, you can accommodate, roll it into equal-sized balls (as large or small as you choose) and put it on a cling film or baking tray that is parchment lined. Refrigerate for an hour.

o   When they're chilling, start to melt the chocolate in a heat-resistant container, either in a microwave or in a glass bowl over a boiling water pan.

o   When melted, allow to cool moderately and cover with a cling film or with a baking sheet.

o   Take the balls from the refrigerator and use a skewer coat in dark chocolate until each ball it is fully coated.

o   Return to a baking tray and then sprinkle each truffle with salted chopped peanuts until coated.

o   Return to the refrigerator for at least an hour to rest before dining.

o   Remove and let it rest for a minute or two until you feed. Enjoy!

8. Brownie Fat Bombs

Servings: 1 | Total time: 45 min

Calories 118 Kcal | Carbs: 2g |Protein: 5g |Fat: 9g

Ingredients

o   Smooth peanut butter 250g

o   Cocoa 65g

o   Zero syrup 2-4 tbsp

o   Coconut oil 2 tbsp

o   Salt ¼ tsp

Steps of preparation

o   Simply transfer all the ingredients to the food processor, rubbing near the bottom, if necessary, until mixed into a dough.

o   While using liquid sweetener or Zero Syrup or a coconut oil, refrigerate dough in refrigerator till the mixture is solid enough to scoop into a little scoop or spoonful of ice cream. Roll in the balls of your perfect size and serve and enjoy!

9. Cheesy Stuffed Mushrooms

Servings: 12 | Total time: 15 min

Calories: 72 Kcal, |Fat: 7g |Protein: 6g | Carbohydrates: 0g Fat: 5g

Ingredients

o   Bacon 225g
o   Mushrooms 12
o   Butter 2 tbsp
o   Cream cheese 200g
o   Finely chopped 3 tbsp chives,
o   Paprika powder 1 tsp
o   Salt and pepper

Steps of preparation

o   Start by preheating the oven to 200 ° F.
o   Now fry the bacon until it becomes really crisp. Enable to cool and afterward toss into the crumbs – save the fat of the bacon.
o   Take the stems from the shrooms and cut them finely. Fry in the bacon fat, add the butter if needed.
o   In a dish, blend the bacon crumbs with the fried mushroom stems and the leftover marinade.
o   Cover each of the mushrooms with a mixture and then bake for 20 minutes until it gets golden brown.

10. Keto Peanut Butter Granola

Servings: 12 | Total time: 40 min

Calories: 338 Kcal, |Fat: 30g |Protein: 9g | Carbohydrates: 9g

Ingredients

o   Almonds 1 1/2 cups
o   Pecans 1 1/2 cups
o   Coconut 1 cup shredded
o   Sunflower seeds 1/4 cup
o   Swerve Sweetener 1/3 cup
o   Vanilla 1/3 cup
o   Peanut butter 1/3 cup
o   Butter 1/4 cup
o   Water 1/4 cup

Steps of preparation

o   Preheat the oven to 300F and line a wide-rimmed baking tray with a parchment paper.
o   Process the almonds and pecans in a processor until they match rough crumbs with some bigger parts. Now transfer them to a large bowl and then mix in a, sunflower seeds, shredded coconut, sweetener and some vanilla extract.
o   Now melt the peanut butter and the butter together in a microwave safe jar.
o   Pour the molten peanut butter mixture over the nut mixture and combine gently,

stirring gently. Stir it in the water. Mixture is going to clump together.

o Now spread mixture uniformly on the prepared lined baking sheet for 30 minutes, by stirring halfway through. Now remove and let it cool off completely.

11. Ketogenic hot caramel chocolate

Servings: 1 | Total time: 6 min

Calories: 144 Kcal, |Fat: 14g |Protein: 14g | Carbohydrates: 4g

Ingredients

o Unsweetened almond milk 1/2 cup
o Heavy whipping cream 2 tbsp
o Cocoa powder 1 tbsp
o Salted caramel collagen 1 to 2 tbsp
o Liquid sweetener
o Whipped cream
o Caramel sauce

Steps of preparation

o Combine almond or the hemp milk and heavy cream in a pan over medium heat. Get it to a boil.

o In a mixer, incorporate the chocolate powder and the collagen. Put in the hot milk and mix until the milk is frothy.

o Top with thinly sweetened ice cream and a caramel sauce to top it off!

12. Ketogenic brownie bark

Servings: 12 | Total time: 45 min

Calories: 98 Kcal, |Fat: 8.3g |Protein: 2.4g | Carbohydrates: 4.3g

Ingredients

o Almond flour 1/2 cup
o Baking powder 1/2 tsp
o Salt 1/4 tsp
o Room temperature 2 leg whites
o Swerve sweetener 1/2 cup
o Cocoa powder 3 tbsp
o Instant coffee 1 tsp
o Butter melted 1/4 cup
o Heavy whipping cream 1 tbsp
o Vanilla 1/2 tsp
o Chocolate chips 1/3 cups

Steps of Preparation

o Start by preheating the oven to 325F and place parchment paper on a baking sheet. Lubricate the parchment paper with oil.

o In a small cup, mix together the flour, baking powder and the salt.

o Mix the egg whites in a large bowl until it becomes foggy. Mix in the sweetener, chocolate powder and some instant coffee until it becomes smooth and then mix in the melted butter, cream and the vanilla.

Mix in a mixture with almond flour until it is well mixed.

o Now spread the batter on the lubricated parchment in a square of around 12 by 12 inches. Sprinkle some chocolate chips.

o Now bake for 18 minutes, until it is puffed and all set. Remove from the oven, turn the oven off and let it cool for 15 minutes.

o Using a sharp knife, cut through 2-inch squares, but do not detach. Return to a warm oven for about 5 to 10 minutes and toast lightly.

o Remove, let it cool fully, then divide into squares.

13. Ketogenic Homemade Nutella

Servings: 6 | Total time: 20 min

Calories: 158 Kcal, |Fat: 18.3g |Protein: 3.3g | Carbohydrates: 18 g

Ingredients

o Hazelnuts toasted 3/4 cup

o Coconut oil 2 to 3 tbsp

o Cocoa powder 2 tbsp

o Powdered swerve sweetener 2 tbsp

o Vanilla extract 1/2 tsp

o Pinch salt

Steps of Preparation

o Grind hazelnuts in a processor until finely ground and starts to clump together.

o Now add two tablespoons oil and keep on grinding until the nuts become smooth out. Add remaining of the ingredients and then blend until well mixed. in case of thick mixture, add one more tablespoon oil.

14. Ketogenic snickerdoodle truffles

Servings: 24 truffles yield | Total time: 20 min

Calories: 150 Kcal, |Fat: 14g |Protein: 3g | Carbohydrates: 13 g

Ingredients

o Almond flour 2 cups

o Swerve 1/2 cup

o Cream of tartar 1 tsp

o Ground cinnamon 1 tsp

o Salt 1/4 tsp

o Butter 6 tbsp

o Vanilla extract 1 tsp

o Swerve 3 tbsp

o Ground cinnamon 1 tsp

Steps of preparation

o In a large bowl, mix together the Swerve, the cream of tartar, the almond flour, cinnamon, and the salt. Now stir in melted butter and some vanilla extract till the dough is combined. Add a tablespoon of water in case of hard dough and stir together.

- Now scoop dough with rounded tablespoon and then squeeze in the palm and hold together, now roll into a ball. Transfer on a waxed paper which is lined on a cookie sheet, and then repeat.
- In a small bowl, mix together the cinnamon and the Swerve. Now roll the truffles in this coating.
- Serve.

15. Chocolate chip keto cookies

Servings: 20 | Total time: 30 min

Calories: 238 kcal | Proteins: 4.3 g | Carbohydrates: 8.18 g | Fat:21.5 g

Ingredients

- Almond flour 1 1/4 cups
- Unsweetened coconut 3/4 cups
- Baking powder 1 tsp
- Salt 1/2 tsp
- Butter softened 1/2 cup
- Swerve sweetener 1/2 cup
- Yacon syrup or molasses 2 tsp
- Vanilla extract 1/2 tsp
- Egg 1 large
- Chocolate chips sugar-free 1 cup

Steps of preparation

- Start by preheating the oven to a temperature of 325F and then line a baking sheet with the parchment paper.

- In a small bowl, mix together some almond flour, baking powder, salt and coconut.
- In a big bowl, add cream butter and the Swerve Sweetener along with molasses. Add in vanilla and egg, beat until well mixed. Now beat in some flour mixture till dough is well mixed completely.
- Mix in some chocolate chips.
- Now shape the dough into small balls and then place them 2 inches apart on the lined baking sheet. Press the ball to a 1/4 inch of thickness.
- Now bake 12 to 15 minutes, till just starts to brown.
- Let cool completely on the pan after removing from oven.
- Serve.

16. Keto Fat Bomb with jam and Peanut butter

Servings: 12 | Total time: 45 min

Calories: 223 kcal | Proteins: 3.8 g | Carbohydrates: 4.5 g | Fat:21.5 g

Ingredients

- Raspberries 3/4 cup
- Water 1/4 cup
- powdered Swerve Sweetener 6 to 8 tbsp
- grass-fed gelatin 1 tsp
- creamy peanut butter 3/4 cup

- o coconut oil 3/4 cup

Steps of preparation

- o Fill a muffin tin with 12 liners of parchment paper.
- o Mix the raspberries and water in a small saucepan. Bring it to a boil and lower the heat and simmer for 5 minutes. Now mash the berries with your fork.
- o Mix in 2 to 4 tbsp of powdered sweetener, based on how sweet you want. Mix in the peanut butter and gelatin and let it cool.
- o Mix peanut butter and the coconut oil in a microwave safe jar. Cook on maximum for 30 to 60 seconds, once it has melted. Whisk the powdered sweetener in 2 to 4 tbsp, depending about how sweet you want it.
- o Partition half of peanut butter mixture into 12 cups and put in the freezer for around 15 minutes. Divide the mixture of raspberry between the cups then top with the remaining mixture of peanut butter.
- o Chill in refrigerator until becomes solid.

17. Classic Blueberry Scones

Servings: 12 | Total time: 40 min

Calories: 223 kcal | Proteins: 5.5 g | Carbohydrates: 7.21 g | Fat:12 g

Ingredients

- o Almond flour 2 cups
- o swerve sweetener 1/3 cup
- o coconut flour 1/4 cup
- o Baking powder 1 tbsp
- o Tsp salt 1/4
- o Eggs 2 large
- o Heavy whipping cream 1/4 cup
- o Vanilla extract 1/2 tsp
- o Fresh blueberries 3/4 cup

Steps of Preparation

- o Preheat the oven to 325F and cover a big baking sheet with a silicone lining or a parchment paper.
- o In a big bowl, mix together the rice, coconut flour, the baking powder, sweetener, and salt.
- o Mix in the eggs, whipped cream and vanilla and combine until the dough starts to combine. Include the blueberries.
- o Assemble the dough together and now place on the prepared baking sheet. Put in a rugged rectangle measuring 10 x 8 inches.
- o Using a sharp, broad knife to break into six squares. Then split each of these squares laterally into the two triangles. Gently raise the scones and then scatter them across the tray.

- Bake for almost 25 minutes until becomes golden brown. Remove it and leave it cool.
- Serve.

18. Chocolate coconut cups

Servings: 20 | Total time: 20 min

Calories: 223 kcal | Proteins: 5.5 g | Carbohydrates: 7.21 g | Fat:12 g

Ingredients

- Coconut butter 1/2 cup
- Kelapo coconut oil 1/2 cup
- Unsweetened coconut 1/2 cup
- Powdered swerve sweetener 3 tbsp
- Ounces cocoa butter 1 & 1/2
- Unsweetened chocolate 1 ounce
- Powdered swerve sweetener 1/4 cup
- Cocoa powder 1/4 cup
- Vanilla extract 1/4 tsp

Steps of preparation

- For candies, cover a mini muffin tray with a 20 mini paper lining.
- Mix coconut butter and the coconut oil in a small saucepan over low flame. Stir until melted and creamy, then mix in the shredded coconut and the sweetener until merged.
- Divide the mixture between the prepared muffin cups and then freeze until solid, for around 30 minutes.

- For chocolate coating, mix cocoa butter and the unsweetened chocolate in a bowl placed on a pan of simmering water. Stir until it has melted.
- Mix in the sifted powdered sweetener and now stir in cocoa powder until smooth.
- Now remove from the heat and whisk in the extract of vanilla.
- Put   chocolate topping over the coconut candies and then let it cook for around 15 minutes.
- Candies can be kept on your kitchen countertop for up to one week.

19. Roll biscotti

Servings: 15 | Total time: 1 hr. 20 min

Calories: 123 kcal | Proteins: 4 g | Carbohydrates: 4 g | Fat:12 g

Ingredients

- Swerve Sweetener 2 tbsp
- Ground cinnamon 1 tsp
- Almond flour Honeyville 2 cups
- Swerve Sweetener 1/3 cup
- Baking powder 1 tsp
- Xanthan gum 1/2 tsp
- Salt 1/4 tsp
- Melted butter 1/4 cup
- Egg 1 large
- Vanilla extract 1 tsp
- Swerve Sweetener 1/4 cup

- Heavy cream 2 tbsp
- Vanilla 1/2 tsp

Steps of preparation

- In a small bowl, combine the sweetener and the cinnamon for filling. Set it apart.
- Preheat the oven to a temperature of 325F, cover the baking sheet with the parchment paper.
- In a big bowl, whisk together the starch, baking powder, the xanthan gum, sweetener, and salt. Stir in 1/4 cup of butter, the egg and the vanilla extract before the dough fits together.
- Turn the dough onto the lined baking sheet and then half it in two. Shape each half into a rectangular shape of around 10 by 4 inches. Making sure the scale and form of both halves are identical.
- Sprinkle with around 2/3 of cinnamon filling. Cover with one of the other parts of the dough, close the seams and then smooth the cover.
- Bake for almost 25 minutes or until gently browned and solid to the touch. Transfer from the oven and spray the remaining melted butter on it, then dust with the leftover cinnamon mixture. Allow it to cool for about 30 minutes and reduce the temperature to 250F.

- Cut log into around 15 slices with sharp knife.
- Place the slices back on the cut-side in the baking sheet and bake for another 15 minutes, then turn over and bake for the next 15 minutes. Turn the oven off and let it stay within until it's cold.

20. Garahm crackers

Servings: 10 | Total time: 1 hr. 5 min

Calories: 156 kcal | Proteins: 5 g | Carbohydrates: 6 g | Fat:13 g

Ingredients

- Almond flour 2 cups
- Swerve brown 1/3 cup
- Cinnamon 2 tsp
- Baking powder 1 tsp
- A pinch of salt
- Egg 1 large
- Butter melted 2 tbsp
- Vanilla extract 1 tsp

Steps of preparation

- Preheat the oven to 300F for crackers.
- In a big cup, stir together flour, cinnamon, baking powder, sweetener, and salt. Stir in egg, melted butter, molasses and vanilla extract before the dough falls together.
- Transform the dough into a wide sheet of parchment paper and pat into a rough

rectangle. Cover with a sheet of parchment. Print out the dough to around 1/8-inch thickness as uniformly as possible.

o   Cut the top of the parchment and now use a sharp knife to rank around 2x2 inches in squares. Move the whole piece of parchment to the baking sheet.

o   Bake for 20 to 30 minutes, until brown and strong. Remove the crackers and let them cool for 30 minutes, then split up along the score. Return to the warm oven if it's so far cooled off, turn it on and adjust the temperature to no higher than 200F). Let it sit for yet another 30 minutes, then cool absolutely.

Chapter 6: Keto Smoothies for women above 50

The ketogenic diet requires a drastic reduction in your carbohydrate consumption and, instead, you get much of your daily intake of calories from fats. Because the keto diet restricts carbohydrates, smoothies that include high-care products such as bananas, yogurt, honey, and milk do not typically work into this form of eating. This could be a matter for those who depend on smoothies for a leisurely and balanced breakfast or a snack. Luckily, there are already some low-carb smoothies and healthy foods for women above 50 that you will appreciate when adopting a keto diet.

1. Ketogenic Berry Smoothie

Servings: 1 | Total time: 1 min

Calories: 254 kcal | Proteins: 2.2 g | Carbohydrates: 5 g | Fat:24 g

Ingredients

o   Ice 2 cups
o   Mixed Berries frozen 1 cup
o   Powdered Fruit Erythritol 1/4 cup
o   Vanilla Collagen 2 scoops
o   Unsweetened Coconut Milk 1 cup

Steps of preparation

o   Transfer all the supplies to the high-speed blender.
o   Then use the "smoothie" mode or mix until it is creamy.

2. Ketogenic Peanut Smoothie

Servings: 1 | Total time: 1 min

Calories: 192 kcal | Proteins: 6 g | Carbohydrates: 8 g | Fat:17 g

Ingredients

o   Milk of choice half cup
o   Peanut butter 1 tbsp
o   Cocoa powder 1 tbsp
o   Peanut butter 1-2 tbsp
o   Avocado 1/4 medium
o   Liquid stevia 1 serving
o   Ice 1/4 cup

Steps of preparation

o   Transfer all the ingredients, besides ice, to a blender or a food processor and blend well.
o   If the smoothie becomes too dense, incorporate enough milk to obtain the perfect consistency. Add any more ice or peanut butter when the smoothie becomes too thin.
o   Transfer in a bottle and drink!

3. Peppermint Milkshake

Servings: 3 | Total time: 10 min

Calories: 198 kcal | Proteins: 10 g | Carbohydrates: 15 g | Fat:20 g

Ingredients

o Highland Milk 2 cups
o Ice Cream Vanilla flavor 1 cup
o Peppermint Extract 2 teaspoon
o Candy Canes Crushed
o Optional Whipped Cream

Steps of preparation

o Transfer all of the ingredients to a blending machine.
o Blend the ingredients.
o Now top with your favorite whipped cream and candy canes.

4. Chia Seed Vanilla Smoothie

Servings: 1 | Total time: 2 min

Calories: 538 kcal | Proteins: 28 g | Carbohydrates: 6 g | Fat:39 g

Ingredients

o Cacao butter 2 tbsp
o Coconut milk 1 cup
o Protein powder 1 scoop
o Coconut oil half tbsp
o Vanilla extract 2 tsp
o Ginger ½ tsp
o Chia seeds 1 tbsp
o Monk fruit sweetener 2 tbsp
o Ice cubes 5-10

Steps of preparation

o Transfer the almond milk and then transfer all the other ingredients.
o Now blend by using a blender for around a minute.
o Now serve and enjoy!

5. Matcha Green Energy Smoothie

Servings: 1 | Total time: 3 min

Calories: 75 kcal | Proteins: 4 g | Carbohydrates: 8 g | Fat:1 g

Ingredients

o Coconut Milk 1 Cup
o Matcha Powder 1 tsp
o Spinach 1 Cup
o Ice Cubes 1 Cup
o Monk fruit 2 tbsp
o Blueberries 1/4 cup
o Whole Almonds 10

Steps of preparation

o Transfer all ingredients in a blender and then blend until it becomes smooth.

6. Almond Ketogenic Milk Avocado Smoothie

Servings: 1 | Total time: 2 min

Calories: 106 kcal | Proteins: 1 g | Carbohydrates: 12 g | Fat:7 g

Ingredients

- o Frozen strawberries 1 lb.
- o Almond Milk 1 half cups
- o Avocado 1 large
- o Powdered Allulose 1/4 cup

Steps of preparation

- o Place all the ingredients in a blender and blend until smooth. Alter sweetener to taste as desired.

7. Ketogenic Vanilla Milkshake

Servings: 1 jar | Total time: 2 min

Calories: 367 kcal | Proteins: 2.8 g | Carbohydrates: 3.1 g | Fat:38 g

Ingredients

- o Unsweetened almond milk ⅔ cup
- o Heavy cream ½ cup
- o Vanilla ½ pod
- o Vanilla extract ½ tsp
- o 5 ice cubes

Steps of preparation

- o Start by cutting the vanilla pod in half.
- o Remove the seed.
- o Move the heavy cream to the pot and introduce the vanilla seeds as well as the scratched-out pod into the heavy cream.
- o Simmer the heavy cream while stirring continuously.

- o Extract the scraped vanilla pods from its heavy cream and apply the infused heavy cream to the container or cup.
- o Ice in the refrigerator until it's cold.
- o Transfer the heavy cream mixture and all the other ingredients to the food processor and mix for approx. 30 seconds.

8. Strawberry Smoothie

Servings: 2 | Total time: 2 min

Calories: 155 kcal | Proteins: 1 g | Carbohydrates: 3. g | Fat:38 g

Ingredients

- o Whipping cream 1/4 cup
- o Almond milk 3/4 cup
- o Granulated stevia/erythritol 2 teaspoons
- o Frozen strawberries 4 ounces
- o Ice half cup
- o Vanilla extract half teaspoon

Steps of preparation

- o Transfer all ingredients into a blender.
- o Blended it and start scraping sides if required
- o Transfer into two glasses to serve.

9. Coconut avocado smoothie

Servings: 2 | Total time: 2 min

Calories: 170 kcal | Proteins: 3 g | Carbohydrates: 1 g | Fat:40 g

Ingredients

- Coconut milk half cup
- Avocado half medium
- Cacao powder 1-2 tablespoons
- Vanilla extract half teaspoon
- Salt of choice
- Erythritol 2-4 tablespoons
- Ice half cup
- Water
- Chia seeds ground

Steps of preparation

- Transfer coconut milk, cacao powder, avocado, vanilla extract, salt, add-ins of choice to a blender sweetener. Blend it well until becomes creamy and smooth.
- Transfer in ice and mix until thick, smooth, and creamy. Enjoy!

10. Peanut Butter with Chocolate Smoothie

Servings: 1 | Total time: 5 min

Calories: 375 kcal | Proteins: 28 g | Carbohydrates: 5 g | Fat:40 g

Ingredients

- Peanut butter 1 teaspoon
- Cocoa powder a pinch
- Heavy cream as required
- almond milk 1 cup
- Sweetener as required
- Sea salt as required

Steps of preparation

- Introduce all ingredients into the blender.
- Mix it until smooth. Add sweetener if desired

11. Green Smoothie

Servings: 1 | Total time: 5 min

Calories: 142 kcal | Proteins: 5 g | Carbohydrates: 16 g | Fat:8 g

Ingredients

- Filtered water 1 cup
- Avocado half
- MCT oil 1 tablespoon
- Organic cucumber half
- Leafy greens 1 large
- Dandelion 1 – 2 leaves
- Parsley 2 tablespoons
- Hemp seeds 2 tablespoons
- 1 lemon juice
- Turmeric powder ¼ teaspoon

Steps of preparation

- Mix all ingredients in a blender until becomes smooth, approximately 1 minute. Serve it cold.

12. Protein Minty Green Smoothie

Servings: 1 | Total time: 5 min

Calories: 293 kcal | Proteins: 28 g | Carbohydrates: 11 g | Fat:15 g

Ingredients

- Avocado half
- Fresh spinach 1 cup
- Sweetleaf 10-12 drops
- Whey protein powder 1 scoop
- Almond milk half cup
- Peppermint extract 1/4 tsp
- 1 cup ice

Steps of preparation

- Transfer avocado, protein powder, milk and spinach in a blender and then blend until it becomes smooth. Now add the peppermint extract, and then ice, and finally blend until it gets thick. Now taste and adjust as desired.

13. Green Low-Carb Smoothie

Servings: 2 | Total time: 5 min

Calories: 168 kcal | Proteins: 6 g | Carbohydrates: 7 g | Fat: 8 g

Ingredients

- Almond milk 1.5 cups
- Spinach 1 oz
- Cucumber 50 grams
- Celery 50 grams
- Avocado 50 grams
- Coconut oil 1 tbsp

- Liquid stevia 10 drops
- Isopure 1 scoop
- Chia seeds half tsp
- Matcha powder 1 tsp

Steps of preparation

- Add almond milk and some spinach to a processor. Mix the spinach for a second to make space for the remainder of the ingredients.
- Simply adding the rest of the ingredients and then blend for around a minute until it gets creamy.
- Incorporate a teaspoon of the matcha powder for additional advantages and a boost of caffeine.
- Mix in a cup and then garnish with chia seeds. Serve and enjoy it.

14. Tropical Pink Smoothie

Servings: 1 | Total time: 5 min

Calories: 402 kcal | Proteins: 24 g | Carbohydrates: 12 g | Fat: 28 g

Ingredients

- Dragon fruit half small
- Honeydew 1 small wedge
- Coconut milk half cup
- Whey protein powder 1 scoop
- Chia seeds 1 tbsp
- Liquid stevia extract 3-6 drops
- Water half cup

Steps of preparation

o Place all ingredients in a blender and mix until smooth. Add the ice after blending

o Use pink or white dragon fruit. Cut it in half and then scoop the meat out.

o Transfer the smoothie into a glass and garnish with scooped dragon fruit and enjoy.

15. Ketogenic Almond Butter Smoothie

Servings: 1 | Total time: 5 min

Calories: 345 kcal | Proteins: 15 g | Carbohydrates: 8 g | Fat: 20 g

Ingredients

o Unsweetened Acai Puree 1 100g Pack

o Unsweetened Almond Milk 3/4 cup

o An Avocado 1/4

o Collagen 3 tbsp

o Coconut Oil 1 tbsp

o Almond Butter 1 tbsp

o Vanilla Extract half tsp

o Liquid Stevia 2 drops

Steps of preparation

o Run the acai puree pack under the lukewarm water few seconds till the puree can be broken into smaller pieces. Now open the pack and transfer the contents into the food blender.

o Transfer the remaining constituents in the blender and then blend until it gets smooth. Now add more water if needed.

o Sprinkle the almond butter around the side of the glass to garnish.

o Enjoy.

16. Ketogenic Blueberry Galaxy Smoothie

Servings: 1 | Total time: 5 min

Calories: 343 kcal | Proteins: 31 g | Carbohydrates: 3 g | Fat: 21 g

Ingredients

o Coconut Milk 1 cup

o Blueberries 1/4 cup

o Vanilla Extract 1 tsp

o MCT Oil 1 tsp

o Protein Powder 30 g

Steps of preparation

o Transfer all the ingredients into a blender.

o Now blend it until it gets smooth.

17. Almond Butter Cinnamon Smoothie

Servings: 1 | Total time: 2 min

Calories: 326 kcal | Proteins: 19 g | Carbohydrates: 11 g | Fat: 27 g

Ingredients

o Nut milk 1 half cups

- Collagen 1 scoop
- Almond butter 2 tbsp
- Golden flax meal 2 tbsp
- Cinnamon ½ tsp
- Liquid stevia 15 drops
- Almond extract 1/8 tsp
- Salt 1/8 tsp

Steps of preparation

- Transfer all the ingredients to a food blender and mix to get a smooth consistency.
- Enjoy.

18. Green Matcha Shake

Servings: 1 | Total time: 5 min

Calories: 334 kcal | Proteins: 19 g | Carbohydrates: 13 g | Fat: 24

Ingredients

- Unsweetened milk 1 cup
- Coconut milk ¼ cup
- Unflavored whey protein 1 scoop
- Matcha oil powder 1 scoop
- Handful spinach 1 large
- Avocado 1 small
- Coconut oil 1 tablespoon
- Ice 1 cup

Steps of preparation

- Transfer all ingredients to a blender and then blend until gets smooth.

- Now garnish with mint leaves and some berries if you want.

19. Ketogenic strawberry smoothie

Servings: 1 | Total time: 2 min

Calories: 149 kcal | Proteins: 6 g | Carbohydrates: 8 g | Fat: 11 g

Ingredients

- Strawberries 1/2 cup
- Coconut milk 1/3 cup
- Water 2/3 cup
- Vanilla extract 1/2 teaspoon

Steps of preparation

- Transfer all of the ingredients in the blender.
- Now blend until it gets smooth.
- Enjoy

20. Ketogenic Berries and Cream smoothie

Servings: 1 | Total time: 5 min

Calories: 549 kcal | Proteins: 10 g | Carbohydrates: 10 g | Fat: 50 g

Ingredients

- Coconut milk 1 cup
- Frozen raspberries ⅓ cup
- Coconut oil 1 tbsp
- Collagen 1 scoop

Steps of preparation

o   Transfer all ingredients and blend until
    gets smooth.
o   Enjoy!

Chapter 7: Gym friendly keto recipes

Appropriate pre and the post-workout treats will help you get through the difficult parts of maintaining keto whenever you're on exercise.

1. Protein Bars

Servings: 18 bars | Time: 1 Hour 15 min

Calories 414 | Total Fat 13 g |Total Carbohydrate 51 g| Protein 25 g

Ingredients

o   Almonds 1 cup
o   Cashews 1 cup
o   Egg white
o   Dates 10 ounces
o   Water 2-4 tbsps.
o   Cinnamon 1 tbsp
o   Unsweetened coconut flakes ¼ cup

Steps of preparation

o   Sheet an 8x8 parchment paper on a plate.
o   Process the peanuts, cashews, cinnamon, and coconut, egg white in your food processor until the nuts have been split down into tiny parts. The "chunkiness" is down to the required flavor.
o   Introduce the pitted dates and then process. Add in the sugar, a single tablespoon at a time, then blend until the mixture holds together. When you pass it to the plate, the paste should be sticky.
o   Flatten it with your fingertips. Freeze for around 1 hour. Cut like the bars.
o   You should pop the bars in your Ziplock bag and then put them inside your exercise bag.

2. Keto Avocado Egg Salad

Servings 4 | Time: 15 min

Calories: 119.0 |Total Fat: 8.7 g |Protein: 7.2 g | Saturated Fat: 1.8 g

Ingredients

o   Large eggs 4
o   Ripe avocado 1
o   Chives 1 handful
o   Parsley 1 handful
o   1 lemon juice
o   Salt and pepper to taste

Steps of preparation

o   Boil the eggs hard and then peel them.
o   Scoop out the avocado in the boats
o   In a medium dish, put the eggs with the avocado and the herbs. Apply the juice of a lemon and the seasoning. Now Mash with a fork.

- o Scoop in avocado the boats
- o Wrap it up in a lunch box or a plastic container.

3. Keto Salmon Cucumber Rollups

Servings 6 | Time: 1 hr.

Calories 111 | Fat 8g | Protein 5g

Ingredients

- o English cucumber 1 long
- o Smoked salmon ½ cup
- o Cream cheese ½ cup

Steps of preparation

- o First, peel the cucumber into 6-inch lengths with a vegetable peeler.
- o Spoon around 1-2 teaspoons of the cream cheese across the length of cucumber.
- o Now Press a piece of smoked salmon to the tip of the cream cheese and curl the cucumber as firmly as feasible.
  - o Secure with the help of a toothpick and roll with a wax paper. It's not going to last long but can remain fresh in a lidded container.

4. Ketogenic Fat Bomb Squares

Servings: 36 squares | Time: 25 min

Calories: 107 kcal | Carbohydrates: 2g | Protein: 2g | Fat: 10g

Ingredients

- o Coconut flakes, unsweetened 4 cups
- o Coconut oil 1 cup
- o Chocolate chips 1 cup
- o Butter ½ cup
- o Sweetener of your choice, 2 tbsp powdered
- o Vanilla 1 tsp

Steps of preparation

- o Melt the coconut oil together with the butter.
- o Incorporate the melted butter and the coconut oil with the chocolate flakes.
- o Put 1 tablespoon of vanilla and blend properly.
- o Put in the sugar and blend.
- o Place the parchment paper in a square skillet and slowly pour into the bottom. Freeze once set up.
- o Melt chocolate chips by placing a glass bowl in a pan of water, even coat.
- o Remove the coconut mixture from the freezer and now coat the top with chocolate, spread on it to make a beautiful, even coat.
- o Freeze it fully.

5. Ketogenic Banana Bread Muffins

Servings 6 | Time: 30 min

Calories 295 | Protein 9.3g | | Fat 27.4g | Total Carbs 7.7g

Ingredients

- Eggs 3 large
- Mashed bananas 1 cups
- Almond butter ½ cup
- Vanilla 1 teaspoon
- Coconut flour ½ cup
- Cinnamon 1 tbsp
- Baking powder 1 tsp
- Baking soda 1 tsp
- Sea salt

Steps of preparation

- Start by pre-heating the oven to 350 F. Grease the pan.
- In a large bowl, combine the eggs, the banana butter, and the vanilla.
- Whisk until it's completely mixed.
- Combine the dry ingredients and mix with a wooden spoon till mixed.
- Spoon the batter in the muffin tins. Bake them for about 15 to 18 minutes.

6. Ketogenic Carmelitas

Servings: 12 | Time 1 hour

Calories: 59 |Carbs: 11g | Protein: 1g Fat: 1g |

Ingredients

- Unsweetened coconut 1 cup
- Sliced almonds 3/4 cup
- Almond flour 1 cup
- Sweetener of your choice ½ cup
- Coconut flour 3 tbsp
- Baking soda ½ tsp
- Salt 1/3 tsp
- Butter, melted ½ cup
- Sugar-free caramel sauce 1 cup
- Chocolate chips 1/3 sugar-free

Steps of preparation

- Preheat the oven to 225F and then grease the 9x9 inch square sheet.
- In a food processor, mix the coconut and the sliced almond. Those are to substitute the oats, so they're going to have to be around the size when you're finished.
- Transfer this to a big bowl of almond flour, coconut flour, baking soda, sweetener, and salt. In the melting butter, stir.
- Press half of the mixture to the base of the baking tray. Bake for 10 minutes.
- Cool thoroughly and prepare the caramel sauce and the chocolate chips.
- Now Spread the caramel sauce and then the chocolate chips. Transfer its other half of the mix to the surface and bake for another 15 minutes.

7. Ketogenic Chipotle Beef Jerky

Servings: 6 | Total Time: 1 hour

Calories 168 |Total Fat 8g |Carbohydrates 1g| Carbohydrates 1g |Protein 25g

Ingredients

- Flank steak 1 ½ lb.
- Soy sauce 1/3 cup
- Liquid smoke 2 tsp
- Chipotle powder 1 tsp
- Chipotle salt ½ tsp
- Chipotle flakes 2 tsp
- Onion powder 1 tsp
- Paprika 1 tsp
- Black pepper

Steps of preparation

- Freeze the flank steak for almost 2 hours to make it easy to slice. Cut in small and thin strips.
- Use the leftover supplies to prepare the marinade. Put the sliced beef, stir to cover, cap, and put in the refrigerator for at least 24 hours.
- Preheat oven to the lowest possible level. Lay the slices of steak on the baking sheet. Bake in the oven with the oven door open slightly. It should require almost 4-6 hours to dry out entirely, and you must turn the meat after every two hours.

8 Keto on The Go Egg Cups

Servings 8 | Time 35 min

Calories: 78kcal | Protein: 6g | Fat: 5g| Carbohydrates: 2g |

Ingredients

- Eggs 12
- Cooked bacon 4 oz
- Cheddar cheese 4 oz
- Sun-dried tomatoes 4 oz

Steps of preparation

- Preheat the oven to 400F
- Put the cupcake liner in the muffin tin
- Crack the egg in each muffin cup and fill it with your desired blend-ins. You can use cheese, sausage, and dried tomatoes. However, you can substitute it with anything you want instead.
- Now Season it.
- Bake for about 15 minutes.

9. Keto post work out shakes

Servings: 2 | Time: 5 min

Calories: 447 |Fat: 42 g |Carbohydrates: 8.5 g | Protein: 21 grams

Ingredients

- Vanilla whey protein 2 scoops
- Almond butter 1 tablespoon
- Avocado 1/2 ripe
- Chia seeds 1 tablespoon
- Full-fat coconut milk 1 cup
- Ice cubes 6

Steps of preparation

o Put all ingredients in a blender and then blend until smooth.

7.10. Keto-Friendly exercise shake

Servings 1 Smoothie | Total Time 6 minutes

Calories 220 kcal | Calories: 220 | Net Carbs: 3 g | Fat: 15 g | Protein: 11 g

Ingredients

o Avocado ½ ripped

o Cocoa Powder 1 tbsp

o Vanilla Almond Milk 1 Cup Unsweetened

o Stevia 1 tsp

o Collagen 1 tbsp

o Cinnamon 1/2 tsp

o Ice Cubes 5-7

Steps of preparation

o Rinse the avocado and then slice it in half. Now put in half the avocado in the blender and then save the remaining for another smoothie.

o Now add the cocoa powder, collagen, cinnamon, stevia, and ice cubes into the blender.

o Now add the almond milk.

o In the end, Blend/pulse until creamy.

o Transfer into a glass and serve.

Conclusion

This book explained keto diet in detail, which is a high-fat, low-carbohydrate diet similar to Atkins & low-carb diets. It involves substantially reducing the consumption of carbohydrates and replacing them with fat. After reading this book, you will several unique concerns and subjects that relate mainly or exclusively to women over 50 on keto diet. There are some key takeaways for women above 50 on keto Diet and the problems one has to be aware of. After reading this book, you will learn some easy, rapid and simple recipes for women above 50. These include the breakfast, lunch and the dinner keto-based recipes, which are low in carbohydrates. This book also presented some delicious snacks and smoothies too. Some exercise and gym friendly recipes are also presented.

CPSIA information can be obtained
at www.ICGtesting.com
Printed in the USA
LVHW021119161120
671799LV00007B/143